LI███████████

Candida albi██████████████████ yeast organism li████████████████ n our lifestyles go ████████████████ ads of antibiotics, oral contraceptives, high-fashion fermented foods such as cheese and alcohol, and sugar and other refined carbohydrates, a Candida overgrowth—candidiasis—signals us that we are asking for trouble . . . and in fact have it.

Candidiasis can depress immune system function and lead to a myriad of health problems, including arthritis, allergies, intestinal malfunction, and may be implicated in birth defects and cancer. Candidiasis can be countered by medical therapy, but the recommendations for diet, healing attitude and lifestyle changes set forth in this insightful, authoritative book are needed for a full return to optimum health.

Shirley Lorenzani has experienced and conquered candidiasis. She is a practicing nutritionist, bringing an unusual awareness of the interdependency of physical, psychological and mental components to her direct, practical approach to the problems Candida presents.

In *Candida: A Twentieth Century Disease*, author Lorenzani clarifies the complications of this diagnostically elusive condition and presents workable solutions which can bring undreamed-of relief to the tens of millions of Americans—as many as one in three—whose health is impaired by candidiasis.

Other Relevant Keats Books

Candida Albicans by Roy Wunderlich, M.D. and Dwight K. Kalita, Ph.D.

The Candida Albicans Yeast-Free Cookbook by Pat Connolly and Associates of the Price-Pottenger Nutrition Foundation

The Famous Bristol Detox Diet for Cancer Patients by Alec Forbes, M.D.

First Edition 1984–85 Yearbook of Nutritional Medicine edited by Jeffrey Bland, Ph.D.

Medical Applications of Clinical Nutrition edited by Jeffrey Bland, Ph.D.

Mental and Elemental Nutrients by Carl C. Pfeiffer, M.D., Ph.D.

The Nutrition Desk Reference by Robert H. Garrison Jr., R.Ph. and Elizabeth Somer, M.A.

Solved: The Riddle of Illness by Stephen E. Langer, M.D.

Your Body Is Your Best Doctor by Melvin Page, D.D.S.

CANDIDA:

A Twentieth Century Disease

by

SHIRLEY S. LORENZANI, Ph.D.

Keats Publishing, Inc.   New Canaan, Connecticut

Candida: A Twentieth Century Disease is not intended as medical advice. Its intention is solely informational and educational. Please consult a medical or health professional should the need for one be indicated. Neither the author nor the publisher has authorized the use of their names or the use of any of the material contained in this book in connection with the sale, promotion or advertising of any product or apparatus. Any such use is strictly unauthorized and in violation of the rights of Shirley S. Lorenzani and Keats Publishing, Inc.

CANDIDA: *A Twentieth Century Disease*

Pivot Original Health Edition
Copyright © 1986 by Shirley S. Lorenzani

Library of Congress Catalog Number: 85-81549

ISBN: 0-87983-375-0

Printed in the United States of America

PIVOT ORIGINAL HEALTH BOOKS are published by

Keats Publishing, Inc.
27 Pine Street (Box 876)
New Canaan, Connecticut 06840

This book is dedicated to
my parents
MILDRED BRUNER STOTT
and
WILLIAM ABDOL STOTT, SR.

These individuals are gratefully acknowledged for their contributions to this book:

Barry Bennett, Ph.D.
Emanuel Cheraskin, M.D., D.M.D.
Pat Connolly
Wayne Dyer, Ph.D.
Werner Erhard
James Fraser
Betty Goldstein
Bill Grover
B.F. Hart, M.D.
Bonnie Jarrett
Bonnie Johnson
Marianne Lucas
W.W. Mittelstadt, M.D., D.O.
Lee Nealey

Bruce Pacetti
Melvin E. Page, D.D.S.
Bernard Palmer
Suzanne M. Peoples, M.D.
Weston A. Price, D.D.S.
Sondra Ray
John-Roger
Roberta Ruggiero
Robert Schuller
R. W. Snow, M.D.
Lendon Smith, M.D.
C. Orian Truss, M.D.
Chris Spoor
Michael Ziff, D.D.S.
Sam Ziff, Ph.D.

CONTENTS

CANDIDA ALBICANS:
Friend or Foe?

THE HUMAN BODY is a wonderful place in which to live. We aren't the only ones who think so. In the intestines, not to speak of the nose, ears, mouth or vagina, over 400 different species of microorganisms eat, sleep, give birth and die.

Humans have an extraordinary relationship with these organisms. Civilizations of them rise or fall when we change our diet. A series of antibiotics profoundly affects the sociopolitical hierarchy in your gut.

Do these organisms profoundly affect you in return? You bet! Chemicals produced by them enter the bloodstream, going everywhere your blood goes. That includes your brain. Some of these chemicals seem to influence thought, foster mood swings and impair memory.

Candida albicans is an eminently powerful microorganism. The fact is, it's innocuous, incapable of causing disease in a healthy human. But then, where is a healthy human these days? Unhealthy humans seem to be the rule rather than the exception, and succumb easily to Candida's chemicals.

Candida is not new. For ages it had barely survived from one generation of human intestines to the next. This century, its number finally came up. Thriving on antibiotic drugs, oral contraceptives and sugar, it couldn't have found a more appropriate time or place to prosper than in the twentieth century U.S.A.

For years Candida had still another advantage—anonymity. Humans were reluctant to report increasing amounts of intestinal gas and bloating. Women assumed vaginal discharge was normal and didn't complain. Most doctors, and even more lay people, did not even know that Candida was around.

Now, Candida has the spotlight. It is the subject of medical seminars, the recipient of research grants. Physicians who are aware of its existence see it frequently.

This book tells the story of Candida: What it is, what it does, how you can know if you "have it," what causes it and how to reverse its overgrowth in your body.

Candida is not cause for panic. Sure, it's serious. Scientists are linking it to AIDS, birth defects and cancer. It's being called the most important medical issue of our time—the twentieth century disease. A prominent University of California immunologist, Alan Levin, recently estimated that one out of every three Americans is being adversely affected by this organism.

So why not panic? Because along with this new perspective on Candida, we're taking a new perspective in viewing ourselves. We no longer see ourselves as helpless victims of disease. More and more people are claiming control of their health. This is reflected in natural food sales, best sellers, fitness club memberships, and healing procedures in which the patient participates.

Symptoms of disease—such as Candida overgrowth—are being recognized as a signal, an important message that something in our lifestyle needs to be altered. When we have made the proper changes, our self-healing mechanisms are free to perform the functions for which they were created.

As an important part of this warning system, Candida albicans is a friend, not an enemy. It signals us when drugs, foods and other forms of distress have weakened our defenses. It is our smoke detector, our burglar alarm, our seat belt buzzer. The signals may be annoying, but the early warning, if heeded, enables us to avoid disaster.

Our old view of disease would have seen Candida as a parasite. We, the humans, would have been the helpless victims of this malicious organism that invaded our bodies, attacked our defenseless tissues. In that context, we were perpetually at war. Every ailment, sign or symptom of illness was an indication of hopelessness in the battle against disease.

Now we know that we are not victims of disease, especially candidiasis. We control our health by what we eat, the drugs we take, the exercise we do or don't do, the thoughts we have. Lifestyle has been the trendy term to use in reference to this collage of what we do. Maybe healthstyle is a more appropriate label for the way we live our lives.

Candida is the barometer *par excellence* of the quality of your healthstyle. Candida overgrowth is saying, "Make some changes fast or worse things are on the way for you! Why don't you reexamine your diet, consider another form of contraception, get off those antibiotics and build your resistance through healthy daily living?"

Serving in this valuable role of health critic, Candida is a loyal member of our internal ecosystem. Not a parasite, it is our symbiont.

Fungi which coexist with other living things—such as humans—are viewed as symbionts if the partnership is of mutual benefit. If you, or people close to you, are suffering with Candida overgrowth, it may be difficult for you to see benefit in the human/Candida relationship. It is there. Although it may look as though Candida is the problem, Candida is merely pointing to the problem.

The problem of unhealthy daily living that Candida exposes is actually an opportunity. It is an opportunity to learn what is really good for you; what sustains and supports, not corrodes and destroys, your health and vitality.

What looks like a breakdown can be a breakthrough, an exciting chance to explore your powerful healing processes.

II FUNGI:
The Third Kingdom

ARE YOU READY for one more indicator that life is becoming increasingly complicated? Remember when it was fairly simple to classify living things? They were either plants or animals. Forget that little system. While we were busy driving to and from work, sorting the laundry and electing presidents, scientists were busy reorganizing our world. Having decided that lots of living things didn't look or act like plants or animals, they came up with some new categories. One of those is fungi, the third kingdom.

Members of the third kingdom include molds, mildews, puffballs, mushrooms, and yeasts. Diverse in complexity and size, they range from single-celled microscopic organisms to giant puffballs that grow up to six feet in diameter. At least 100,000 different species have been identified with thousands more discovered each year. Mycologists, scientists who specialize in the study of fungi, tell us that these forms of life are difficult to classify. Although some of them may resemble plants, they contain no chlorophyll and cannot make their own food. Like

5

us, the animals, they use oxygen and have a nucleus within each cell.

Fungi may be difficult to classify, but they are not difficult to find. They are amazing in their ability to thrive in cool to tropical climates. Some prefer water while others choose moist shady soil. Manure is the favorite habitat for some species while others revel in dead leaves, fruit or leftover food. Colorful, smelly mildews grow on shoes, books and clothing during periods of high humidity. Other fungi grow on bread and vegetables. Molds which grow on living plants are considered diseases, such as those which affect cereal grains and other food crops.

You are almost certain to have encountered members of the third kingdom in your bathroom because shower tile grout is a hospitable locale. To the other extreme, you have probably chosen fungi in the most elegant restaurants—mushrooms in wine sauce or delicate truffles.

Actually, you have encountered fascinating fungi at much closer range than your shower or dinner plate. Try between your toes. That is usually *Trichophytum rubrum*. *Pityrosporum ovale* prefers the oily parts of the skin, like the area around the nose. The population there may be up to one-half million organisms per square centimeter. *Candida parapsilosis* and *Candida guilliermondii* are not so particular about where they live, just as long as it is on skin. Four different species have been identified as normal inhabitants of the external ear. And that's just the *outside* of your body! Mouth, intestines and genitals all provide comfortable homes for many other species of fungi.

Is it out of malicious intentions that fungi have established colonies in your most private places? No. Nature doesn't usually have it planned that way. Fungi aren't on your scalp to cause dandruff.

They are just recycling some of the debris found in that vicinity. And so it goes on other parts of your body, and on your damp books, and on your bathroom floor.

Fungi perform an invaluable planetary task of helping along the process of decay. Without them, we would be wading through mounds of plant and animal remains, the wind wafting chicken feathers that had been around since the Paleozoic era into our field of vision. The grand finale of this fungal-induced decay is that nutrients get returned to the soil, enabling life to begin anew.

Fungi do not acquire food by ingesting it as animals do. Their cell walls are too rigid to allow the entry of even microscopic particles. Instead, they secrete potent enzymes which break down the material from which they obtain nutrients. The wood or other organic material, predigested into smaller molecules, is then absorbed into the filaments of the fungus. This unique process allows a soft, delicate fungus to penetrate the hardest of woods. It simply digests its way into its source of food.

Fossil remains suggest that fungi have been digesting and recycling our planet for quite a while. Paleontological studies indicate that fungi may have existed in the pre-Cambrian period. That could be 1500 million years ago. Undisputed fossil remains date fungi from the Devonian period, making them at least 405 million years old.

Humans used the life processes of yeasts and molds long before they were understood by modern science. Fermentation, the process by which yeast converts carbohydrates into other substances, probably has enhanced our food supply since prehistoric times.

It is not difficult to imagine the discovery of leavening in the preparation of grains. People observed that when grains were crushed, mixed with water and left in a warm place, interesting and desirable changes occurred. The grains, moist and warm, were a perfect growth medium for yeast from the air. These yeasts landed on the grains and began recycling the sugar they found there to carbon dioxide and water. Bubbles of carbon dioxide gas caused the grains to rise. Heating the raised grains in the sun or in primitive ovens killed the yeast and prevented further fermentation. The alcohol produced during fermentation evaporated in the baking process, leaving our prehistoric ancestors with sandwich potential.

The process of baking was refined without being understood until the 1800s, when several scientists almost simultaneously demonstrated that yeasts are living organisms that decompose sugars to create fermented foods. Louis Pasteur furnished irrefutable demonstrations of the role of living microorganisms in fermentation. The mysterious transformations resulting in beer, wine, bread, cheese, vinegar and sauerkraut were then understood.

Today, baking is far removed from the primitive procedures of our ancestors. Baker's yeast, a commercially prepared leavening organism, has replaced wild yeast from the air. Bread dough is usually a mixture of flour, water or milk, salt, a concentrated sugar and yeast, with the flour providing only a small amount of the sugar needed for fermentation. The chemical process, however, has always remained the same:

Yeast + Glucose ———> Carbon Dioxide + Alcohol
            (Sugar)

In the baking industry, it is the carbon dioxide in this reaction which produces the desired result— leavened bread. In the wine and beer industry, the alcohol portion of the reaction is the desired end.

Evidence exists that professional wine and beer making was established 3,000 years before Christ.

Egyptian documents described the production and consumption of beer in 2,500 B.C. Records indicate its use in China in 2,300 B.C. An Assyrian tablet dated at 2,000 B.C. declares that Noah was able to tolerate all those animals so well because he had a stash of his favorite mash aboard the ark!

Fermentation of any fruit juice with a high sugar content produces an alcoholic beverage. The most commonly used is grape juice, with fermentation beginning as soon as the grape skin is broken. European wineries allow the wild yeast naturally growing on the grape to perform this fermentation process. American wine makers usually seed their vats with a specific strain of yeast. As fermentation proceeds, the vats bubble with carbon dioxide. Sugar is being consumed in this reaction and ethyl alcohol is produced. When the alcohol level nears 14 percent, the yeast cells begin to die. Their death brings a halt to the fermentation process. The raw wine is then poured into containers where it sits for a month or more. Dead yeast cells settle to the bottom before the wine is bottled.

Beer is produced in much the same way. Malt, derived from the seeds of barley plants, is used instead of grape juice and prepared brewer's yeast ferments the grain into alcohol. In the production of all alcohol, producers are careful to limit the supply of oxygen during fermentation. When oxygen is abundant, yeasts ferment, using their aerobic (oxygen) cycle. In this type of reaction, no alcohol is produced, only carbon dioxide and water.

All liquor is made by fermentation in a limited amount of air. Yeast converts corn mash into bourbon, fruit juices into brandy, rye grains into rye whiskey, sugar cane into rum, barley malt into Scotch, and potatoes into vodka.

To accompany these liquid ferments, the dairy industry provides solid ferments in the form of cheese. You can thank the blue-green mold *Penicillium* for the memorable flavor of Camembert and Roquefort cheeses: the same mold that produces the antibiotic penicillin. Yeast-fermented milks such as kefir, koumiss, or matzoon are popular beverages in Eastern European countries. The unique textures and flavors of butter, buttermilk, cheeses, yogurt, and other dairy products are due in part to the types of microorganisms, i.e., fungi or bacteria, used in fermentation and other processes of production.

Vegetables and their juices are fermented to make such items as sauerkraut, pickles, and ripe olives. The vinegar used to preserve foods such as these is usually a ferment of wine or cider. In one vinegar-making process, fruit juice is fermented by *Saccharomyces cervisiae*, a brewer's yeast. When the alcohol level reaches 10 percent, the liquid is inoculated with a bacterial species which converts the alcohol into acetic acid, the chemist's name for vinegar.

Not all fungi are employed by the food and beverage industry. Many yeasts and molds work for major drug companies. This liaison began in the 1940s when mold-produced chemicals and antibiotics ushered in "The Golden Age of Chemotherapy."

The destruction of one living thing by another is the magic of antibiotic drugs. The name is derived from the term antibiosis. Antibiosis abounds in the arena of living organisms. From the biggest creatures to microorganisms, living things survive by killing and eating other organisms. Our present use of the term antibiotic is more specific, however. A chemical substance or metabolic product of a microorganism that is detrimental to other microorganisms is an official antibiotic.

Long before scientists became specific in their understanding of antibiosis, the process was being used in health care. The Chinese began experimenting with antibiotics 2,500 years ago, discovering that the moldy curd of soybeans had curative properties. They used it regularly to treat boils, carbuncles and other infections.

The modern era of antibiotics took off in 1928 with, in retrospect, what looks like an obvious observation made by Sir Alexander Fleming, an English bacteriologist. Fleming noticed that one of his laboratory colonies of staphylococcal bacteria was contaminated with a blue-green mold. Contamination by airborne spores was a common source of aggravation to most scientists. Fleming, however, took the time to look carefully at what was happening as a result of the mold invasion. The bacteria showed signs of destruction! He later interpreted this destruction as the result of antibacterial action of the product from the living mold. The end product was penicillin.

The potential for saving lives from infectious, bacteria-based diseases was dramatic. It would take time, however for this potential to be realized. Fleming and other scientists worked with subcultures of his original mold for almost fifteen years. Chemists, bacteriologists, industrialists and government agencies were enlisted to begin cultivating molds and bacteria with the goal of mass-producing penicillin. During 1943, the production of this drug increased from less than 100 million units in January to ninety times that amount by December. Never in its history had the U.S. government taken such an avid interest in a medical discovery. Generous financial support was given to drug companies and millions of dollars went into the cultivation, harvesting and purification of the new wonder drug.

Many previously fatal diseases responded almost miraculously to penicillin—pneumonia, meningitis, diphtheria, syphilis and strep infections. These successes motivated the search for other antibiotics to deal with resistant organisms such as the tubercle bacillus. Soon streptomycin, another product of a mold, was literally unearthed by a soil microbiologist. More was to follow in the form of tetracycline, erythromicin, ampicillin and amoxicillin.

The importance of mold- and bacteria- produced antibiotics cannot be overstated. Before antibiotics, the U.S. death rate from *Pneumococcus*-induced pneumonia ranged from 20 percent to 85 percent. After antibiotics the rate fell to 5 percent. Death from chronic infection of heart valves has plummeted from 100 percent to 5 percent. Epidemics of spinal meningitis once left death statistics of 20 percent to 90 percent. Antibiotic therapy has lowered that figure to 2 percent.

Fungi have also participated actively in the prevention of disease by digesting and decomposing excrement. In this role, they are employed by sewage treatment plants. Many types of microorganisms engage in rapidly decomposing garbage, fecal waste and other forms of organic debris. Scientific sewage disposal, with appropriately used bacteria and fungi, has enabled us to speed up nature's processes and to keep pace with the staggering volume of waste generated by urban living.

The powerful chemicals produced by fungi are cultivated commercially for many other uses. The yeast *Citromyces* ferments citric acid from sugar. Industry uses citric acid in foods and in blueprinting. Oxalic acid is a ferment of the yeast *Aspergillus niger*. The leather and textile industries use oxalic acid to make dyes and condition raw materials. Other microbial products include enzymes used in removing stains from clothes.

Clearly, the third kingdom is of great benefit to mankind. This is not to say, however, that the products and activities of fungi are always considered friendly. Farmers, for example, do not always agree with the timing at which molds and mildews recycle their plants into the soil. Biblical farmers refer to crop diseases such as cereal rusts as the result of offensive acts against God. Currently, millions of dollars in crop losses each year are attributed to fungi. Chestnut tree blight, Dutch elm disease and apple scab are caused by sac fungi at work.

Fungi growth on food crops not only brings disease to the planet, but also to those who eat it. Ergot is a disease of cereal grains and is also the source of LSD. Eating ergot-infested grains can result in ergotism, characterized by hallucinations.

Historians wonder if ergotism played a leading role in the dramatic Salem witch trials in 1692. A season of cool, moist weather, perfect for ergot growth, was recorded in that year. Convulsive ergotism, a result of eating fungus-infested grain, may have produced hallucinations and bizarre behavior among adolescents in this New England colony. Similar erratic behavior by "bewitched" children was documented in other parts of Essex County, Massachusetts and Fairfield County, Connecticut, where the weather was the same as in Salem.

If you are of Irish origin, your ancestors probably experienced the profound influence of *Phytophthora infestans*. Having a preference for potatoes and finding the weather of 1845–1847 particularly favorable, this fungus organism decimated Ireland's potato crop. Food shortages resulted in perhaps a million deaths on the usually verdant Isle and the emigration of hundreds of thousands of Irish people to America.

III CANDIDIASIS:
Chronic Yeast Infection

WITH FUNGI FAMILIES living in or on almost every living thing, one might expect to find a few on the human animal. Actually, over 300 different types of yeasts and fungi have been identified as normal flora of human skin. And then there are the warm, moist internal environments—mouth, esophagus, intestines and vagina—that make cozy havens for other species.

These organisms are not there to cause disease. In fact, medical mycologists, scientists who specialize in fungi-related health problems, tell us that there are no inherently pathogenic yeasts. These organisms are incapable of producing disease in a healthy human. In the healthy individual, they are probably performing a valuable ecological role.

This is not to say that yeasts are entirely nonviolent. Their violence, however, is usually directed at other yeasts. With so many species in limited spaces, there is fierce competition for food and shelter. Once a strain has set up housekeeping, it produces antibiotics to suppress the growth of competitors, maintaining a balance among species. The fungi are also in competition with bacterial flora, vying for territory.

Of all the strains of yeast which have homesteaded in humans, the most prolific is *Candida albicans*. Its favorite residence is the gastrointestinal tract, from mouth to rectum. The genitourinary tract and female genitals are also preferred areas. Preference for individuals doesn't seem too specific. Any human will do. A study by Chew and Theus in 1967 showed that 100 percent of adults studied were supporting colonies of Candida albicans. Another study by Axelson in 1976 revealed antibodies to Candida in 163 of 169 adults. Cultures of mucosal surfaces, delayed skin tests, antibody levels all suggest the same. Virtually all humans are in partnership with Candida albicans.

This partnership began early for most of us. Infants usually encounter Candida in the birth canal, and thus bring it with them out into the world. If not, Mother shares it in her loving kisses and tender caresses, because Candida lives in the mouth and on the hands of most adults. By the age of six months, 90 percent of all babies have a positive skin test to Candida albicans.

It is amazing how well-designed the healthy human host is for self defense against overgrowth of such microorganisms as Candida albicans. The very dryness of our skin is protection against external yeast overgrowth. Sophisticated internal systems draw on resources such as specialized blood cells to engulf invading organisms and maintain an ecological balance.

Not so long ago, these blood cells with names like B and T cells, and the lymphatic organs—spleen, thymus and lymph nodes—were defined as the immune system. These components were thought to be almost solely responsible for internally defending the human organism against disease. Rallying this system was known as "the immune response."

Today scientists are taking a closer, or broader, look at the immune system. They are seeing that all parts of the human body participate in its defense. Each sense—vision, hearing, touch, smell—signals danger in its unique way. Does that not make eyes, ears, skin and nose parts of the immune system?

Less obvious immune functions are performed by the digestive system. Digestion and absorption of nutrients come under the category of provisions, essential to any defense department. Teeth, gum, esophagus, intestines, pancreas, liver and salivary glands all perform vital roles in the processing of food. Carbohydrates, fats, proteins, vitamins, minerals and enzymes are converted into a state that can be used to nurture, repair and empower every participant in the system.

Transporting the provisions to the front lines—the front lines being almost everywhere—is the circulatory system. This network is clearly an essential participant in "Project Defense." Arteries and veins, our human highways, crisscross, shortcut and streamline their way to every tissue and cell. Their traveler is our sustaining liquid, the blood. Blood transports nutrients and provisions and provides transportation to troops. These particular defenders called phagocytes and antibodies are alert to attack and disarm invaders such as yeasts and their toxic byproducts.

On the return trip, the blood carries away waste products which otherwise would clutter up and poison cells and tissues. This brings another system into the immunology department—the urinary system. Excreting wastes, maintaining water, salt and acid balance, the kidneys are at the command post of this division. Filtering, selectively discarding and reabsorbing substances, the kidneys are designed to produce, with incredible precision, urine of a specific color, transparency and weight. The thirst mechanism by which the body ensures a steady supply of water is a result of communication from the kidneys.

Chemical messengers handle many communications in the defense department. Like homing pigeons, these chemicals are released in one area of the body and travel through the blood to a predesignated target organ. That organ then responds to chemically encoded instructions. The tissues that release these carrier chemicals directly into the bloodstream are the endocrine glands and their chemicals are called hormones.

Endocrine glands and their hormones include the adrenal glands, (which produce cortisone), sex hormones and a host of other powerful messengers. The pancreas contributes insulin, whispering to every cell the password which allows the entrance of blood sugar through the cellular membrane. The pituitary gland, gonads and thyroid all add to the flow their special chemicals, affecting changes and maintaining equilibrium in such areas as basal metabolism, growth, menstrual cycles, distribution of fat and even the frequency of urination.

Our muscles and skeletal system, nervous system, every gland and organ are engaged in maintaining stability. This special balance, constant equilibrium, is called homeostasis.

When stability is continuously upset and the body becomes too exhausted to maintain its steady state, disease overcomes the human defenses. Arthritis, multiple sclerosis, depression, diabetes, heart disease, even cancer can be seen as the result of an exhausted immune system. Yeast overgrowth is clearly the outcome of a defense department crippled by frequent upsets.

None other than the father of modern medicine himself, Hippocrates, was the first to record Candida albicans overgrowth in debilitated patients. Way back in 400 B.C. he wrote of white patches growing in the mouth and throat of weak and sick individuals. Today we refer to this type of Candida albicans overgrowth as "thrush."

Although thrush, oral candidiasis, can occur in any age group, we usually think of it as a children's disease. For hundreds of years, textbooks on pediatrics have described the milk-curd-like colonies in the mouths of newborn babies. Associated with diaper rash, another form of candidiasis, oral thrush is common in babies less than a month old. Pregnant women often have a mild case of vaginal candidiasis, also called moniliasis or monilia, which the baby picks up during birth. The infant's immune system is usually able to win the battle against Candida albicans rather quickly. Thrush is rare in infants over one month old.

Candidiasis does not seem to be rare in their mothers. Female anatomy can provide hospitable habitat for yeast overgrowth. Combined with a defective immune system, it is the perfect environment for yeast organisms to proliferate in wild abandon. When this occurs, there is usually a thick, milky discharge. Gray-white patches, similar in appearance to the curdlike thrush patches in the mouths of infants, can be seen on the surfaces of the vagina. Itching, burning, soreness and even ulcers can occur in the vaginal area.

It's not a long trip for yeast organisms to travel from the vagina to the rectum, nor is it a one-way street. Yeast colonies in the intestines can quite easily send pioneers in the direction of the vagina. Intestinal candidiasis can produce what doctors call "irritable bowel syndrome." Patients know it as constipation and/or diarrhea, cramping, bloating and a noisy growling. Sometimes the stool may contain blood or mucus and chronic constipation may produce hemorrhoids. Rectal itching or tingling may be a nuisance.

Many digestive problems may be a direct result of yeast overgrowth. Heartburn and sour stomach are linked with Candida colonies in the esophagus, the tube connecting the mouth to the stomach. Defective opening and closing of the valve between the esophagus and stomach is often a source of burning and pain. Is this condition, labeled "hiatus hernia," connected with yeast overgrowth? Could be.

Yeast is easy to see in the adult mouth. Open wide. Oral thrush coats the tongue with a creamy white curdlike film. Patches of yeast growth may also spot the gums and corners of the mouth. Gums may be sore and bleed easily. The tongue and gums may tingle and feel tender and irritated.

Given that the mouth is connected to the rectum, the thighbone to the kneebone, and the ear to the toe, it is easy to see how adventurous yeast organisms move from one part of the body to another. Colonies may begin in the mouth or vagina, but if the immune system is not on guard, Candida can go virtually anywhere.

Studies reveal that this yeast organism is present in almost all lung conditions. Bronchial candidiasis is a form of chronic bronchitis. It is characterized by coughing, with sputum, rales, and a thickening of the bronchial tubes. In advanced cases, the small curdlike yeast patches are visible, growing on the bronchial tree.

Do the toxins released by these yeast organisms create an extremely sensitive respiratory system? Could breathing problems, usually regarded as allergies, be a result of yeast overgrowth? All of the classic allergy symptoms are common in candi-diasis—sneezing, runny nose, stuffiness, post-nasal drip, cough and asthma. The mucous membranes of the respiratory tract from nose to lungs may become irritated by continuous exposure to yeast or its tox-ins. Irritation can lead to infection by other organ-isms, viral or bacterial. Then the label changes from candidiasis to sinusitis, bronchitis, sore throat, a cold or pneumonia.

How many recurring urinary tract infections may be coupled with yeast overgrowth? The urinary sys-tem, the kidneys, ureters and bladder can be havens for Candida albicans. When yeast infects the outer end of the urethra, common when yeast is next door in the vagina, irritation results in urgency, burning and frequent urination. In some cases, little balls, made of Candida and other yeasts, have been found in the urinary tract. It is easy to see how such clumps of Candida could obstruct the tubes used to transport urine.

Candida can grow on heart valves and arteries, or brain tissue or between your toes. Its influence is not limited to areas where it lives. Toxins produced by this yeast enter the blood stream and thus float to all tissues supplied by blood—and that means just about everywhere. The variety of symptoms reported by candidiasis patients, and the disappearance of those symptoms when an anti-yeast health program is followed, suggests that any organ, gland or tissue can be affected by yeast or its by-products.

The brain, complex in its circuitry of neurotrans-mitters and chemical receptors, appears to be dra-matically affected by candidiasis. Memory loss, mood swings and inability to concentrate can be signals of yeast toxicity or overgrowth. A feeling of fogginess, absence of mental clarity and disorientation is common. Depression, frustration and anxiety are reported by many patients.

The senses—sight, smell, hearing, taste, touch—can also change during candidiasis. Sometimes a salty or metallic taste is reported. Vision may be blurred and night blindness may develop. Hearing loss, ringing noises and acute physical sensitivity have all been logged. Clumsiness, a lack of eye-body coordination, is common and numbness in hands and feet can limit the sense of touch.

Apparently, many subtle biochemical aberrations result from candidiasis. These aberrations include the inability of hormones to function normally. Menstrual cycles may become irregular or temporarily disappear. Weight goes up and down like a seesaw. Fluid retention and puffiness in women is evident, especially during premenstrual days. There may be an inability to respond fully during sexual experiences or a total loss of interest in sex.

Do yeast toxins affect the environment around joints, producing symptoms that are often labeled "arthritis"? Joint pain and stiffness often subside with the remission of yeast overgrowth.

When candidiasis disappears, food and chemical sensitivities often disappear. Perfumes, exhaust and chemical emissions from synthetic upholstery, clothing and carpets can present problems during yeast overgrowth. Even health-sustaining foods such as fresh vegetables and whole grains may evoke unpleasant reactions. Scientists think that the waste products from the yeast cells and other Candida-produced chemicals act as toxins to the human body, overwhelming its defenses and setting the stage for allergic reactions to materials which otherwise would not produce reactions. About eighty different yeast toxins have been identified.

Other symptoms of Candida takeover include headaches, lethargy, fatigue, acne, hives, psoriasis, eczema, muscle pain, hypoglycemia (low blood sugar), hypothyroidism (low thyroid) and multiple endocrine disorders.

Are you beginning to get the picture? When the immune system has been crippled by frequent upsets, Candida or its toxins can go almost anywhere and do almost anything.

These toxins can include a chemical called acetaldehyde. This substance is very much like formaldehyde—that's embalming fluid. Like other Candida-produced toxins, acetaldehyde can literally poison every system in the body.

IV
Causes of Candidiasis

YEAST ORGANISMS are incapable of causing disease in a healthy person. For any part of the human body to succumb to yeast, stress must occur on a regular basis. Stress upsets our internal harmony. It disturbs homeostasis, our naturally balanced state.

Where do we find stress? Is it out there in the world, lurking on the job, in traffic, waiting at home? No, stress is always an inside job. It is our personal reaction to events, places and people.

Stress is also a response to poor food choices, inadequate circulation, environmental toxins and hormone imbalances. Drugs, designed to relieve stress and cure disease, often create new stress. The stress caused by drugs is called "side effects" and can, like all other forms of stress, weaken the immune system and lead to yeast overgrowth.

Let's examine several areas in which we often experience stress and see how they lead to Candidiasis.

DIET

Not so many years ago eating rarely caused stress. Most people on the planet ate locally grown, whole, natural vegetables, grains, protein and fruits in season. Preservatives weren't added to foods. Dyes were not deemed necessary. Sugar and other refined sweets were too expensive for the average person to eat daily so desserts were not part of the meal. They were saved for holiday feasts. Overeating was also reserved for holidays and did not occur nightly in front of a television set.

"Oh, come on," you say. "When did humans last show such dietary wisdom? Maybe during biblical times, wandering in the desert."

It may be surprising, but some cultures in the twentieth century have been virtually sugar-free and nongluttonous. These cultures were studied in the 1930s by a dental researcher named Weston A. Price. After he retired from a life of dentistry, Dr. Price traveled the globe in search of large groups of people in excellent health. He found them on every continent: the Masai in Africa, Peruvian Indians high in the Andes, South Sea Islanders, Australian Aborigines, American Eskimos, Swiss in the Lowenthal Valley, New Zealand's Maoris. These people had immune systems of such strength that cavities only rarely occurred in their teeth. The major degenerative diseases of our society—arthritis, cancer, heart disease, diabetes—were practically nonexistent.

Dr. Price observed that the diets of these healthy cultures had a common denominator. Concentrated sweets were not on the table. Sugar, honey, molasses, syrup—none of these foods were used daily. Sweets appeared only on holidays and special celebrations. Members of these cultures who had given up the traditional way of eating and switched to sugary, refined foods were easily identified. In the absence of dentists (previously there had been no need for this profession) black stubbed smiles identified the more modern consumer. Rotting teeth preceded hemorrhoids, arthritis, even birth deformities that had occurred only occasionally in these societies.

Dr. Price speculated that the eating of sugar somehow changed the level of minerals in the body. When minerals were not functioning normally, body chemistry could not work to maintain health.

Another dentist, Dr. Melvin E. Page, decided to investigate exactly what effect concentrated sweet foods had on mineral levels. For several years, he observed thousands of patients, looking for a link between diet and health. Calculating the levels of minerals floating in the blood, he eventually came upon an exciting discovery. When sweets are consumed, the calcium and phosphorus levels in the blood change, often dramatically. These shifts are very stressful to the human body.

Minerals are a vital part of the body's chemical and electrical phenomena. Calcium and phosphorus, only two of many, are like keys, turning on the ignition of various glands, organs and processes. When minerals are not present or cannot work, important functions are impaired. Glands don't put out quite enough hormones, blood sugar remains too high or too low, the liver cannot release stored energy fast enough to prevent fatigue. Since minerals run the body, their ability to perform is critical to health. Sweets affect that ability.

At the Page Clinic, Dr. Page saw the often serious results of regular sugar consumption. His laboratory testing of patients with major health problems revealed that blood mineral levels had been drastically altered. Immune systems had gradually succumbed to chronic disease. Part of the healing process involved avoiding sweet foods and reestablishing mineral levels.

Other studies by equally prominent researchers have pointed accusing fingers at sweets. Neutrophils are the most numerous type of white blood cells. Their special talent is engulfing infectious organisms. Neutrophils do their best work when blood sugar levels are neither too high or too low. In other words, homeostasis helps white blood cells do their job. When blood sugar climbs too high or drops too low, as it often does after the consumption of sugar, honey or even orange juice and apple juice, neutrophils appear almost paralyzed. It is then that infectious organisms can have a heyday.

The evidence consistently reveals that most people with Candida-related health problems have habitually eaten sweets. Although the immune system can be damaged by other forms of stress, sweets are frequently part of the picture.

It is no coincidence that Candida overgrowth is the twentieth century disease and sugar is the twentieth century food. The average American gets the sugar fix at the rate of 120 pounds per year. That works out to two apple pies per capita per day! Most people get their sugar neatly hidden away in catsup, salad dressings, cookies, ice cream, gooey pastries and candies. Others, purists so to speak, prefer their sugar in the more natural state, but still concentrated and stressful—honey, molasses, syrups. Even the sugar in fruit juice, dried fruits and fresh fruits is sometimes too rich for the blood.

Years ago, *Lancet*, one of the world's most respected medical journals, reported a study showing that apple juice produced erratic blood sugar levels in young men who had no history of diabetes. The conclusion of this study was that drinking or eating concentrated sweets separated from the natural fiber of the whole food leads to "disturbed glucose homeostasis."

When glucose, or blood sugar, remains too high and the body can no longer lower it effectively, the condition is labeled diabetes. People with diabetes are especially prone to Candida overgrowth. The blood cells which defend against invading organisms are semiparalyzed when blood sugar is too high. Furthermore, yeast cells thrive on sugar—blood sugar, table sugar, fruit sugar, honey sugar, syrup sugar.

While sugar doesn't do much for the human organism, except thrill our taste buds, it is the food that allows Candida to grow and multiply in great health. Candida albicans and other yeasts grow in all sugars, including fruit, and multiply rapidly in fruit juice. Even freshly squeezed orange juice has been found to contain Candida albicans. Sweet foods that have been stored are even more likely to harbor colonies of Candida and other yeasts. Starchy foods, like potatoes and rice, also provide a perfect environment for yeasts and molds. After grains and potatoes are cooked, yeasts and molds can easily thrive in the moist surroundings and live on the sugar contained in the starch. For this reason, eating leftover starchy foods is not always a good idea. Freshly cooked starchy foods, eaten in moderation, are not usually a problem, but leftovers can be a source of yeasts and molds.

Leftovers are not healthful for other reasons. When foods are stored or reheated, they lose many nutrients. Vitamins, when exposed to heat and light, often undergo destructive chemical changes. Vitamin C is well known for its vanishing act. Let's look at what happens to the vitamin C in cooked potatoes. All our freshly cooked potatoes are a respectable source of vitamin C. Yet, when baked potatoes sit on a steam table for only one-half hour, they lose 34 percent of this nutrient. After forty-five minutes, the loss increases to 59 percent. Obviously, eating overcooked, leftover food is not the best way to get adequate nutrients.

Speaking of nutrients, that's another reason to avoid sugars. Sugars contain such small amounts of vitamins and minerals that they are often referred to by nutritionists as "dead food." Unlike nutrient-rich foods such as broccoli and potatoes, sugars are poverty-stricken. Providing only calories in the form of carbohydrates, sugar lacks vitamins A, B, C, D, E and the full spectrum of minerals needed to support human life. When people satisfy their hunger with sugars, all they get are empty calories.

It is clear that any variety of sugar is destructive to health in several ways:

1. Sugar causes changes in the ability of minerals to function normally, thus shutting down or altering important chemical reactions.
2. Sugar provides almost no vitamins and minerals, earning the label "dead food."
3. Sugars feed yeasts, such as Candida albicans.

Sugars may be the major stress food, but other foods can also upset homeostasis and feed yeasts. Dairy products, milk and cheeses, are not digested well by many adults. Dairy allergies are common and milk sugar, called lactose, can be processed by the body into a sugar that will feed yeasts.

Clinical research at the Page Clinic has shown that alcoholic drinks and caffeine are also stressful substances. While they may not directly encourage yeast growth, they may weaken the body's defenses against Candida.

DRUGS AND YEAST

The real story of the American drug culture is not only that of cocaine, heroin and marijuana, but also the story of 3 billion prescriptions annually and massive consumption of over-the-counter drugs. Approximately 75 million Americans take one or more drugs regularly. About 10 million are on drugs for high blood pressure. At least 5 million regularly consume mild tranquilizers. Aspirin and aspirin-containing compounds are staples in the diet of over 15 million people. Market analysts predict the pharmaceutical industry will get even bigger as drug sales double in the 1980s.

Peering into this pharmacopoeia is like peering into Pandora's box. Looking beyond the obvious benefits, we can see side effects, adverse reactions and dependency addictions. Even more insidious is the tendency of the user to think that the disease process is halted merely because a symptom is being suppressed.

This is not to say that drugs can not be beneficial. At their best, they assist the body's natural mechanisms of healing and restoration. While drugs never cure a disease, they can definitely contribute to a total scheme of healing. Many times, however, that healing scheme would occur quite naturally without the use of a single drug.

When most drugs are prescribed, the doctor is keenly aware that the patient is taking part in an experiment. Drugs have multiple actions, not just one effect. Which effect will predominate in this particular person? And what about allergies, inherited sensitivities and metabolic peculiarities?

One of the largest books on the shelf assists physicians in monitoring these human chemistry experiments. *The Physicians' Desk Reference* lists most of the drugs available in the United States, their commonly prescribed use, contraindications, side effects and adverse reactions. But this book is not a crystal ball. Predictability is limited, even with familiar well-established products, and with new or experimental drugs. Such was the case with the first use of broad-spectrum antibiotics in the late 1940s.

Doctors enthusiastically prescribed these "miracle drugs" to cure pneumonia and other infectious diseases. But a drastic increase in diarrhea and vaginitis accompanied the cure. Astute physicians theorized that the drugs killed bacteria indiscriminately— menacing and friendly alike. This allowed competitive yeast organisms to grow wild, causing gas, bloating, diarrhea and/or constipation, and vaginal itching and discharge.

Although Candida albicans overgrowth has been recorded since the time of Hippocrates, the use of antibiotics has made Candidiasis a common disease. Medical statistics show that before antibiotics were introduced in 1947, only one out of every four vaginal infections was due to Candida. Today, Candida is the cause of nine out of ten such infections.

After years of observation, scientists have concluded that antibiotics or antimicrobial drugs promote yeast infections in four ways:

1. With the destruction of certain microorganisms, vacancies in our internal real estate are created. In these empty spaces, yeasts can proliferate and settle.
2. The bacteria killed by antibiotics often compete with Candida, vying for food as well as space. With the competition dead, Candida thrives easily.
3. Many antibiotics, such as penicillin, tetracycline or streptomycin, directly stimu-

late yeast growth. In a sense, Candida eats these drugs and finds them nourishing. In some circumstances, stimulation of Candida growth after intensive antibiotic therapy has led to fatal complications.

4. Decomposing bacteria can also stimulate and feed Candida. The bacteria killed by antibiotic drugs becomes more food for the yeasts.

The wide variety of antibiotic drugs currently available includes penicillin, tetracycline, streptomycin, ampicillin, amoxicillin, erythromycin, Keflex, Ceclor, Bactrim and Septra.

Antibiotics are not the only drugs that encourage yeast growth. Birth control pills are also known to greatly accelerate the spread of yeast. The two hormones present in most birth control pills are estrogen and progesterone. During the normal menstrual cycle, a woman produces estrogen daily. Progesterone, however, is barely produced during the days between the menstrual period and ovulation at midcycle.

When a woman is pregnant or on the pill, progesterone is being supplied to her tissues continuously. It is the progesterone that somehow stimulates yeast growth. Studies show that about 35 percent of pregnant women and those on birth control pills develop yeast vaginitis. It has also been observed that nonpregnant, nonpill users with chronic yeast infections have a flare-up of symptoms during the two weeks prior to their period. This coincides with the stepped up progesterone released between ovulation and the monthly period. So progesterone is thought to cause changes in the mucous membrane of the vagina. These changes encourage yeasts, which are always present, to multiply. The result is usually vaginitis, with associated symptoms of depression, fatigue and irritability.

Any drug that suppresses the immune system will encourage yeast growth. Certain drugs are specifically designed to shut down the body's defense mechanisms. These include steroids such as cortisone and prednisone. Drugs used in cancer chemotherapy depress the immune response and thus encourage yeast growth. Certain drugs used in the treatment of arthritis also have an anti-immune, pro-yeast side effect.

Many drugs interfere with the ability to use vitamins and minerals. In this way they create nutrient deficiencies, which in turn increase susceptibility to yeast overgrowth. Some drugs absorb nutrients. Other drugs may alter a vitamin or mineral so that the body can no longer use it. Laxatives frequently cause calcium and vitamin D losses. Mineral oil reduces the absorption of vitamins A, D and K. Questran, a cholesterol-lowering agent, can impair the absorption of folic acid. Antacids such as Maalox adversely affect calcium use. Tagamet and slow-release potassium drugs such as Slow-K can reduce B12 absorption.

It is now common knowledge that oral contraceptives create the need for additional vitamin B6 and folic acid. Are you aware that antibiotics call for additional vitamin B2, vitamin C and calcium? Anti-inflammatory drugs, even the lowly aspirin, increase the body's need for folic acid, vitamin C and iron.

Vitamins most commonly depleted by drugs appear to be B6, B12 and folate. Minerals routinely thwarted are potassium, magnesium and calcium. These vitamins and minerals are not merely supporting actors in the drama of human life. They are the stars of our body chemistry. If they are upstaged repeatedly by drugs, the show can barely go on.

Drugs are sometimes lifesaving. Often they provide almost immediate relief from pain. But all too frequently, their prolonged use does not support good health. Since stress of all kinds is thought to lower resistance to disease, any drug which creates more stress than relief will weaken the body's natural immunity to Candida. In this way, many drugs other than the ones cited here, indirectly encourage candidiasis.

GLANDULAR IMBALANCES

The human body is magnificently managed by the endocrine glands. Endocrine means that these glands secrete hormones directly into the bloodstream. The sweat glands and salivary glands do not qualify as endocrine glands because their secretions are not released into the blood.

What are the endocrine glands that produce hormones? There is the *pituitary* gland, about the size of a pea, tucked into a bony nook under the brain. It is well protected there in the center of the head. Nature's infinite wisdom seems to have been at work again, for maximum security is appropriate for this gland. It has been called the master gland, the "queen" gland, and is often described as the conductor of the body's glandular symphony.

The pituitary gland is actually two separate organs; the front lobe is called the anterior pituitary and the portion in the rear is called the posterior pituitary. Each of these two glands produces very important chemical messengers.

The anterior pituitary puts out chemicals that say "Grow!" Many extremely large individuals, notably circus giants, owe their size distinction to a highly overactive anterior pituitary, working overtime to produce excessive growth hormones. Dwarfs, on the contrary, are often the result of an underactive anterior pituitary. Scientists have used this understanding of the anterior pituitary to crossbreed animals. The dachschund dog, dwarfed by an underactive anterior pituitary, is a classic example.

Newborn babies get growth hormone in mother's milk. The production of that milk is stimulated by prolactin, another hormone from the anterior pituitary. This amazing chemical, prolactin, not only gets the milk ready, but is also thought to stimulate motherly love. Animal experiments with prolactin suggest that it somehow inspires affection toward offspring. Other anterior pituitary hormones which are thought to influence disposition and attitude include ACTH, adrenocorticotropic hormone.

The posterior pituitary gland secretes hormones which affect the work of the kidneys. These hormones cause the kidneys to concentrate urine. When there are not enough of the hormones, the kidneys make diluted instead of concentrated urine. The result is frequent urination.

Posterior pituitary hormones also dictate weight distribution. Excess weight below the waist usually indicates low levels of these hormones. Women evidence this in a double hip or bulging thigh just below the hip joint. The weight which accumulates around the middle in the shape of a spare tire is referred to by endocrinologists as the "pituitary girdle."

Another gland whose hormone output is known to influence body weight is the thyroid gland. Nestling against the windpipe, this butterfly-shaped organ releases chemicals which determine the speed at which body chemistry operates. Do you know anyone who rushes about frantically, has a ravenous capacity for food, and is prone to high blood pressure and rapid heartbeat? Those are some of the consequences of a thyroid gland too generous with its chemicals. The normal amount of thyroid hormone produced in one day is minute—$\frac{1}{2800}$ of an ounce per day. More than this amount can lead to the symptoms described above. Less than this amount can result in fatigue, sluggish behavior, lower than normal body temperature and weight gain.

Hyperthyroidism (overactive thyroid) and hypothyroidism (underactive thyroid) can exist on a scale of slight to extreme and are thought to play a significant role in many common health problems. For over fifty years, Broda Barnes, M.D., Ph.D., conducted clinical research into the role of thyroid hormones. He maintained that hypothyroidism is pandemic and that lack of adequate thyroid hormones circulating in the bloodstream is a major factor in cardiovascular disease, menstrual problems and digestive complaints. His theories and observations have recently been presented in a book, *Solved: the Riddle of Illness,* by Stephen E. Langer, M.D. Doctors Langer and Barnes suggest that sex, emotions, blood sugar levels, weight, heart, arteries and your immune system rely on thyroid hormones to stay healthy.

Alongside the thyroid gland are four smaller glands. These *parathyroids* are no larger than grains of rice, yet their hormones perform a big job: they regulate the level of calcium in the blood.

We have plenty of calcium stored in our bodies, more than any other mineral, and the bulk of it goes into bones and teeth. Did you know that calcium is needed in soft tissues as well? As it travels along in the bloodstream it helps maintain the acid/alkaline balance in the blood. It is an essential element in blood clotting after a cut or injury. On a cellular level, calcium escorts nutrients in and out of the cell walls. It assists in our utilization of iron, aids in nerve transmission. In muscle tissue, calcium helps the tissues contract. Since the heart is a muscle, it is obvious that calcium is important.

If calcium is important, the parathyroid glands are very important. Without their hormones, calcium would not be on the scene to perform its duties. When the blood calcium levels drop too low, the parathyroid glands secrete chemicals that bring calcium out of storage depots and put it where it is needed.

Perched atop the kidneys are two glandular dynamos called the *adrenals*. Adrenaline, the "fight or flight" hormone secreted by these glands, shifts our bodies into emergency gear. Its presence in the bloodstream enables a 100-pound mother to lift a several ton car off her child and athletes to come up with a final burst to cross the finish line. In such emergencies, adrenaline is often released at ten times the normal rate. It causes the heart to pump faster, the lungs to take in more oxygen and the blood sugar to rise. Adrenaline also speeds up the clotting time of blood, just in case we're cut during the emergency. It dilates the pupils, raises blood pressure, tones up the heart muscles and moves sugar stored in the liver out into the bloodstream. The adrenal glands are clearly our emergency kit.

The shell of the adrenal glands, called the *adrenal cortex*, makes a different set of chemicals. These hormones handle the routine, nonemergency chores. They stimulate the sex glands, manage mineral levels in the blood, help the kidneys do their work, keep muscles ready to respond and regulate blood sugar levels.

The *thymus* gland, located just above and in front of the heart, has recently been scrutinized by immunologists. This little gland has a big job. It manufactures lymphocytes, specialized blood cells which are the officers of the body's defense forces. Called

T cells, they are thought to control other blood cells by commanding them to destroy bacteria and kill other foreign invaders in the body. The thymus gland might be seen as the West Point of the body's defense department.

As most people age, their thymus gland diminishes in size. An adult usually has a much smaller thymus than a child has. For years, scientists assumed this was normal. Now, there is evidence that a normal healthy adult retains a large thymus. A shrinking thymus seems to be the result of steady and extreme stress. Stress from environmental poisons, junk food, insufficient rest and exercise, emotional upsets and lack of self-love can all shrink the thymus.

The *pancreas* is found in the upper part of the abdomen, just below the heart. Insulin, its special product, is a chemical which floats in the bloodstream to the liver and muscles, where it changes excess blood sugar into a form of sugar that can be stored for later energy needs. This stored sugar is called glycogen. As insulin is carried by the blood to all the cells and tissues, it converts blood sugar into a form that can pass through the membrane of each cell. This enables blood sugar to be used as fuel for the important work going on within the cell.

Too much or too little insulin can result in health problems. When too much insulin is produced, too much sugar is removed from the blood. This leaves a person feeling weak, often dizzy, ravenously hungry, and with exaggerated mood swings that range from giddy hyperactivity to tearful depression.

Too little insulin production is termed diabetes. This is characterized by too much sugar in the bloodstream, because the insulin is insufficient or incapable of removing it for storage or use by the cells.

Both high and low blood sugar levels are crippling to the immune system. Neutrophils, the most plentiful type of white blood cells, are capable of engulfing infectious organisms and are among the body's most important guardians against infection. Experiments have shown that these neutrophils do their best work in blood which has neither too much nor too little blood sugar. This means that blood sugar levels which are either too low or too high weaken neutrophil activity and give foreign organisms a chance to thrive and multiply. These organisms include Candida albicans.

The sex glands, *testes* and *ovaries*, produce chemicals that have effects far beyond the sexual arena. Their vital hormones influence hair growth, personality and overall wellbeing. Both sexes produce estrogen and testosterone, although testosterone is usually termed the male hormone and estrogen the female one.

Males naturally produce more testosterone than do females. Either sex, however, can produce too much of this potent chemical. A person who produces excess testosterone is termed andric. An andric personality is usually in overdrive. Andric men are frequently bald, and andrics of both sexes are more subject to ulcers, heart disease, circulation problems and cancer.

Gynics are those who produce an excess amount of estrogen. This personality type is submissive, with little ambition or assertiveness. Signs commonly associated with too much estrogen are low blood pressure and weight distributed primarily in the lower half of the body.

The *pineal* gland is located within the brain. Little is known about its role in health and disease. It is thought to secrete chemicals that restrain growth and sexual development, working as a counterbalance to the sex glands.

It appears that all the endocrine glands work in tandem. One compensates for another's underactivity by becoming overactive. When ongoing stress offers no relief for the underactive and overactive glands, signs and symptoms of disease promptly appear. The immune system becomes impaired by a myriad of glandular malfunctions. In this context, Candida albicans finds fertile ground to flourish.

CIRCULATION AND CANDIDA

In the mid-nineteenth century, Andrew Taylor Still, M.D. guaranteed himself a place in the history of medical ideas. He said, "The rule of the artery is supreme."

What does this mean? It means that your health depends on the health of your arteries. Without a healthy blood supply, vibrant health is not likely to exist. More specifically, the rule of the artery means that any organ or part of the body can be healthy only if it receives a rich arterial blood flow.

Blood is busy doing more than filling up the space in arteries and veins. It transports life-sustaining material to our cells. Water, oxygen, vitamins, minerals, hormones, glucose and amino acids cannot be delivered without blood flow. Blood also sweeps away cellular debris from the cells, waste products, such as carbon dioxide, lactic acid and urea.

Equally important, blood defends us against foreign organisms. Pathogens, bacteria, viruses and yeasts are held in check by specialized blood cells that engulf and destroy such invaders.

Blood is also our heat distributor. Heat generated by the internal combustion within us is absorbed by the blood. Then it moves around the body to maintain an equal distribution of warmth. One symptom of poor blood flow is cold hands or feet. Without an adequate blood flow, not enough heat is delivered to the ends of the body.

Within the blood are unique cells to handle each function. Red blood cells, viewed from the side, look like little dumbbells. Their most important component, hemoglobin, links with oxygen in the lungs and goes on a one-way trip to the cells. At the cellular depot, carbon dioxide joins hemoglobin for its ride back to the lungs.

White blood cells participate in a process called phagocytosis. This term (from the Greek word *phagein*, meaning to eat) describes the ability of these cells to race to a site of danger, surround the intruding organism and then release powerful enzymes which digest the captured victim. Bacteria, viruses and yeasts which manage to invade through a break in the skin, pass through the filtering hairs of the nose and ears or sneak in with food and survive the stomach acid bath. Ultimately they are met in the blood by one more line of defense—these mighty white blood cells.

If all the blood cells are adequately supplied and arteries deliver an abundance of blood to the tissues, immunity and health are available. When blood supply is less than ideal, so are immunity and health. Tissues then suffer from nutrient deficiencies and unremoved debris forms toxic wastes. Without the oxygen delivered by arterial blood, human cells either suffocate or barely subsist. In territory undefended by white blood cells, foreign pathogens find it easy to do their damage and proliferate.

Fungi and yeast overgrowth have long been linked with inadequate circulation. Physicians scrutinize fingernails and toenails for fungi and yeast, knowing that their presence indicates circulatory problems. When yeast growth is present, the nail appears thickened and there is tissue destruction beneath the nail.

It seems reasonable that yeasts find a hospitable haven in tissues or organs that are poorly supplied with blood. While human cells are crippled by lack of oxygen, yeast cells are not. They can be either aerobic (oxygen-using) or anaerobic (nonoxygen-using). Because of this dual capacity, yeast cells can flourish while human cells are gasping for oxygen. When inadequate blood flow also limits the activity of white blood cells, yeast cells can operate unchecked.

What restricts blood flow and creates a favorable milieu for yeast overgrowth? Biofeedback has clearly demonstrated that tension closes down circulation. When thoughts are shifted from anxious to calm, skin temperature immediately rises. This, of course, indicates increased blood flow.

Numerous studies have shown that hardening of the arteries, arteriosclerosis, affects people of all ages. Autopsies of young American soldiers in the Korean War revealed arteriosclerosis even in the healthiest of our young men. Medical school research has found this disease process active in children only two years old. Each twentieth century stress—most modern food, cigarettes, drugs and alcohol, environmental toxins, lack of exercise, worry and anxiety—has been cited as responsible for the rampant arterial disease process.

Candida, the twentieth century disease, thrives on each human stress factor. It especially thrives as a result of stress which culminates in poor circulation of the blood.

ENVIRONMENTAL TOXINS

Environmental toxin is a nebulous term. A substance that is not even mildly irritating to one person may be toxic or poisonous to another. An extremely debilitated individual, whose immune system barely functions, may experience many common chemicals as enemies. Carpet dyes, cleaning fluid residues, synthetic fabrics, wallpaper glue, linoleum floors, formica cabinets, newspaper ink—are all potential poisons to the sensitive "universal reactor." Indeed, these people seem to react adversely to almost everything in their environment. It is no surprise that they see themselves as victims of the twentieth century.

Man-made chemicals are not the only substances that cause problems. Many toxins are naturally occurring elements, trace minerals from the earth's crust.

Lead is one of these toxins. Over the past few centuries, more and more lead has been released into the environment. Smelters send lead into the atmosphere of industrial areas. Automobile exhaust pipes spew it into parking lots and along highways and streets. Foods grown near industrial smelters or busy highways bring lead to the dinner table. How does it get into the drinking water? Soft water, more acidic than hard water, leaches lead from lead plumbing. Tap water in soft water regions is often contaminated. Other sources include cigarettes, lead-based paint, and pottery glazes.

When lead accumulates in the human body, it interferes with normal body chemistry. A wide spectrum of symptoms appear. Headaches, depression, emotional instability, restlessness, diarrhea, constipation, impaired kidney function, fatigue and gout may develop. Children often experience hyperactivity, learning disabilities, temper tantrums, speech disturbances, seizures and clumsiness. Very young children may exhibit mental retardation.

Mercury, another heavy metal known to be extremely toxic, has frequently made front page headlines. In the 1950s, Japan's Minamata Bay captured the attention of environmentally conscious world citizens when 121 persons died or were disabled after consuming fish from their local waters. Waste containing methyl mercury from a plastics factory had been dumped into the bay.

When seed grain treated with mercury-based fungicide is eaten rather than planted, disaster is guaranteed. Iraq has recorded three such incidents. In 1956, 100 cases of mercury poisoning from seed grain were recorded. In 1960, poisoned bread affected 1,022 people. A world record of mercury poisoning was set in 1972 when Iraq reported 6,350 hospital admissions and 459 deaths. All the classic symptoms of mercury intoxication were present: numbness and tingling of extremities, tremor of hands and unsteady walking.

The United States made mercurial news in 1969 when, in New Mexico, a family of nine butchered and ate hogs that had eaten mercury-treated seed grain. Within weeks, three of the family members suffered derangement of the spinal cord and brain. After an eight-month coma, one girl awoke blind and unable to talk. One young female could walk and talk only with great effort. Her younger brother fell into a four-month state of unconsciousness.

Such dramatic incidents have focused attention on other sources of mercury. Experts pointed to coal burning, batteries, mercury vapor lamps, accidental breaking of thermometer and barometer bulbs, and mercurious medications, such as calomel, as potential hazards to health.

In their careful search for possible mercury sources, guess where most sleuths failed to look? In our mouths! That silver compound filling the holes in most of our teeth is approximately 50 percent mercury.

How did a toxic metal such as mercury become an accepted component in dental fillings? Amidst great controversy, and that controversy is continuing.

Arguments for and against mercury fillings began as early as 1833. Increased sugar consumption was resulting in more holes in teeth. Gold was then the preferred substance of repair, but its disadvantage was obvious. While sugar, with its resultant cavities, was priced for most everyone to afford, gold was not. The time was right for a more economical means of repairing rotting teeth.

Dental entrepreneurs, not licensed dentists, first introduced mercury fillings in New York City in 1833. Professional dentists rose in outrage to protest the use of a compound they claimed was poisonous and would result in gum disease and other ills. The American Society of Dental Surgeons denounced silver-mercury fillings as "hurtful both to the tooth and all parts of the mouth." Members pledged not to use mercury in treating their patients.

Dictates of principles also included principles of economics. More and more dentists quietly turned to mercury amalgams as an affordable alternative to gold. As time went on, these dentists organized to argue that mercury fillings were actually safe as well as inexpensive.

The safety of mercury fillings has, however, never been clearly established. There is an impressive and steadily increasing collection of scientific research showing that the mercury in dental fillings leaks into the teeth, gums, and air in the mouth. Then it may be swallowed, inhaled and absorbed into the bloodstream.

So what? Minute quantities of mercury leaking steadily into the human body. What harm can that do?

Let's take it from the top—the brain. Research has shown that mercury penetrates the blood-brain barrier, a thin membranous tissue that filters many harmful substances that can otherwise enter the brain through the blood. Mercury passes through the filter. All mercury compounds damage the brain. Some cause structural damage. Others alter brain chemistry. If massive amounts of mercury poisoning result in tremors, loss of hearing and vision, and impaired muscle coordination, might not small amounts of ongoing mercury poisoning instigate less obvious damage to the central and peripheral nervous system?

If blood carries mercury to the brain, that means it's going almost everywhere else in the body. Blood tranports mercury to the heart, where it has been shown to interfere with normal cardiac functions. On to the kidneys, mercury has been linked with the destruction of kidney cells and loss of protein into the urine. Massive edema, or swelling, results from heavy mercury exposure.

What about those important endocrine glands, chemical factories whose products profoundly affect the way we look, think and perform? Are endocrine glands harmed by mercury?

We know that mercury accumulates in these glands. Certain glands, such as the pituitary and thyroid, seem to have a special affinity for mercury. Studies of mercury concentration show that the pituitary and thyroid tissues have much higher concentrations than the brain, liver or kidneys.

Animal studies reveal that mercury poisoning dramatically reduces sexual activity by indirectly interfering with hormone production and utilization. Might subtle mercury toxicity affect humans, lowering libido and sexual energy?

What about the blood itself? Does mercury do any

damage to the medium that transports it around the body?

Many animal studies have also shown that mercury damages blood cells that would normally provide immunity against disease. As a recent human study illustrates, this damage also occurs in people. David W. Eggleston, D.D.S. wrote in *The Journal of Prosthetic Dentistry* that he measured the level of T-lymphocytes, commanding officers of the immune system in the blood, before and after he removed mercury amalgam fillings. After the fillings were removed, the number of these specialized blood cells increased by a healthy 55.3 percent. To confirm his suspicions, he reinserted the mercury fillings. T-lymphocyte levels immediately dropped again. Apparently mercury amalgam fillings adversely influence the body's basic immunity to disease.

What do lead or mercury toxicity and exposure to other potentially harmful chemicals have to do with Candida albicans overgrowth? The health of the brain, efficient kidney and heart functions, productive endocrine glands and specialized blood cells are all required for optimum health. If the activities of any of these are continuously compromised by toxic metals slowly and steadily entering the blood stream, foreign organisms, such as Candida, may find it easy to flourish.

PSYCHONEUROIMMUNOLOGY

i can show you love and hate
and the future
dreaming side by side
in a cell
in the little cells where
matter is so fine it merges
into spirit
    DON MARQUIS
    Archy's Life of Mehitabel

It is not a new idea that emotions affect health. Nor does it take a scholarly scientist to reach that conclusion. Your great-grandmother knew about the importance of attitude.

For years, doctors have pointed to emotions as a component in such diseases as asthma, ulcers and colitis. Now, many clinicians are seeing all disease processes—cancer, arthritis, diabetes, chronic headaches, high blood pressure—as having emotional attitude assistance.

In 1984 the American Heart Association met in Miami, Florida. One of the topics of discussion was the prevention of recurring heart attacks. These specialists offered a piece of advice to people who have already experienced one heart attack. How to avoid another one: Watch your diet? No, although that is important. Get regular exercise? That's good, but the cardiologists didn't think that was the most important element in preventing future heart attacks. What did they suggest? Letting go of impatience and anger.

Notice that the advice is to "let go." Nobody said, "don't have." Feelings of anger, fear, worry, impatience, even hate, come to most of us. Trouble really brews when we harbor and hang on to these feelings.

Do you know the type that gets into a traffic jam on the way to work and spends the rest of the day reliving the agonizing experience with everyone in the office? Over and over you hear about the good-ole-days before freeways, the oppressive heat at that hour of the morning, the economics of wasted gasoline, and the ignorance of traffic engineers and city planners. Soon the totality of the twentieth century is at fault. Beneath all the rhetoric is anger, impatience and resentment, repeatedly circulating and growing in intensity. The traffic jam has now been cleared for eight hours, the planet has moved to an entirely new position in the solar system but this character refuses to budge.

When one chooses to remain stuck in guilt, anger, fear, worry, hate or resentment, one is inviting disease. These emotions are themselves dis-ease. Prolong them long enough and they are transformed into frown wrinkles or tension headaches. Let them eat away at you too long and they become ulcers, holes eaten into the stomach lining by the acid which normally digests only your food, not you. Stay "uptight" long after the actual experience is past and rigidity in joints and muscles may appear. Call that arthritis. Refuse to let go of attitudes and emotions that do not nourish your wellbeing. Let them ferment and expand. Constipation, colitis and bloating may be your reward.

An avalanche of studies during the past ten years has confirmed the link between attitudes and ailments. Scientists are now studying animals and humans to see exactly how prolonged stressful emotions can irritate the nervous system, imbalance the endocrine system, and paralyze the body's powerful immune system. Terms for this new science include psychobiology, mood neurobiology, and psychoneuroimmunology.

This new science asserts that destructive disease processes can be set into motion by emotional disturbances. Researchers are now uncovering how the body converts attitudes and emotions into biological change and chemical aberrations.

Once the disease process is firmly entrenched, attitudes of despair and defeat can find extremely fertile ground. When one is in pain or sluggish with constant fatigue, inertia invites more of the same. More resentment, more worry, more fear. "Will I ever feel good again?" "What did I do to deserve this?" "Will the pain ever go away?" Doubt, guilt and confusion simmer and seethe in a brain that is often malfunctioning as a result of abnormal body chemistry.

Our language often contributes to a sense of defeat. People who are experiencing health problems are usually referred to as "victims." Newspaper headlines and media reports broadcast the helpless state of diseased individuals. "Victim of Heart Attack Survives Surgery"; "Stroke Victim Resumes Activities."

Is there any power in the position of victim? Carelessly, we give diseased people who are in great need of inspiration, empowerment and strength a label that implies helplessness, lack of responsibility, and defeat. Even more disastrous, diseased people apply the victim label to themselves, acquiescing to the idea that they have been attacked, invaded and marauded by a force more powerful than themselves. They don't consider that their emotions, diet, lack of exercise, relationships, tension or inadequate rest and relaxation could have had anything to do with the development of health problems. After all, they are victims. The victim stance implies that one never had and does not presently have a choice.

Many twentieth century residents believe that health is not a realistic choice. We live in an era during which diabetes, cancer and heart disease are common. Constipation, fatigue, headaches, sinusitis and gastric distress are considered normal. Who but a Pollyanna expects to be pain-free and radiant with energy after the age of twenty-eight?

Many psychologists, including Wayne Dyer, Ph.D., bestselling author of many self-help books, say that expectations determine much of our health. If you expect to begin irreversibly breaking down at twenty-eight, that's probably what you'll do. If you get up in the morning, experience a sensation of tingling in your throat and declare, "I'm coming down with a cold today," that little tingle will most likely blossom into a stuffy nose, allover aches, and fever by nightfall.

The Bible states, "it is done unto you as you believe." The implications here are profound. If one believes that the disease process is irreversible, for that person, it is. If one believes and steadily sees himself as having been attacked, a helpless victim, destined to suffer, maybe one's immune system responds, or does not respond, accordingly.

The importance of psychoneuroimmunology in relation to Candida albicans is significant. What we are observing is an organism incapable of causing disease in a healthy human. This innocuous organism is creating an epidemic of gigantic proportions. Are we contributing to this epidemic by expecting every germ, parasite, fungus and microscopic organism to overwhelm us? Are we awaiting invasion and ultimate defeat from a hostile world of little critters?

Once ill, do we expect to remain so? Is disease, rather than health, our expected birthright? Have we programmed ourselves to expect bloating, constipation, fatigue, memory loss, loss of libido and menstrual irregularities as part of an aging process that progresses rapidly after twenty? Many people are learning to live with these symptoms of candidiasis, expecting more of the same, unaware that health is available, often on a level they have never known before.

V DIAGNOSING CANDIDIASIS

DIAGNOSIS OF CANDIDIASIS is not a do-it-yourself project. An experienced physician is invaluable in diagnosing and guiding one through the recovery process.

Some physicians feel that laboratory tests are not very helpful in making a diagnosis. These doctors rely on a thorough health history combined with a physical examination. If yeast overgrowth is suspected, a trial of anti-yeast medication and a diet such as outlined in this book is prescribed. If the patient improves on this anti-Candida regimen, it is assumed that yeast overgrowth is or was occurring.

Other physicians prefer laboratory testing as part of the diagnostic procedure. These tests may include cultures of fungus from various areas of the body: nose, throat, rectum, genitalia, under the breasts, skin lesions and armpits.

Another diagnostic tool is a blood test for antibodies. Many labs refer to this test as the Candida Albicans Multi-Immuno Assay.

Some physicians simply study matter from the patient's body under a microscope. Fungi can be detected immediately.

Urine can be tested for the presence of yeast or its by-products. This is an economical and quick procedure.

Researchers are developing improved techniques for making a definitive diagnosis of Candida overgrowth before treatment is begun. At present, however, most physicians will rely on a combination of diagnostic testing and a therapeutic trial of diet and medication.

COMMON SIGNALS OF CANDIDA OVERGROWTH

Gastrointestinal system
chronic heartburn
gastritis
colitis
distension and bloating
gas
indigestion
belching
constipation
diarrhea
rectal itching
hemorrhoids
abdominal pain
mucus in stools

Ears
recurring infections
pain
deafness
fluid in ears

Skin
itching
rashes
psoriasis
dry
scaly
acne

Eyes
spots in vision
burning
tearing
failing vision
blurred vision
erratic vision
chronic inflammation
night blindness

Mouth and throat
sore or bleeding gums
white patches
sore or dry throat
dry mouth
blisters
rash
bad breath
cough

Muscular skeletal system
muscle aches and pains
muscle weakness
muscle paralysis
joint pains
joint stiffness
joint swelling or arthritis

Nose and sinuses
nasal congestion and
   stuffiness
postnasal drip
itching

Lungs and chest
pain and tightness
wheezing or shortness of
   breath
cough

Urinary system
recurring kidney and
   bladder infections
cystitis
urethritis
urinary frequency
burning on urination
urgency to urinate

Generalized
fatigue
increased body hair
loss of body hair
numbness and tingling
weight gain
weight loss
loss of balance and/or
   dizziness
poor coordination
insomnia
excessive sleepiness
overeating
loss of appetite

Women
vaginal burning or itching
vaginal discharge
endometriosis
menstrual cramping
failure to menstruate
too frequent periods

extremely heavy flow
scant menstrual flow
premenstrual depression
premenstrual anxiety

"Allergic" symptoms
hay fever
chronic sinusitis
hives
asthma
food and chemical
   sensitivities

Cardiovascular system
mitral valve prolapse
poor circulation—cold
   hands and/or feet

Sexual
impotence
loss of interest in sex

Men
prostatitis

Emotional/mental nervous
   system
extreme ups and downs in
   moods
irritability
jittery behavior
inability to concentrate
sudden mood swings
poor memory
depression
headaches
lethargy
agitation
"foggy," "spacey"

CANDIDA: A TWENTIETH CENTURY DISEASE

Common yeast-related problems of children

thrush
diaper rash
colic
irritability
recurring ear infections
hyperactivity
learning difficulties
short attention span
nasal congestion
chronic cough
wheezing
headache
digestive problems
constipation
diarrhea
gas and bloating
craving for sweets
mood swings

Diseases thought to be related to or affected by Candida albicans yeast

allergies to chemicals and foods
athlete's foot, ringworm, jock itch and other fungus infections of nails or skin
Crohn's disease
Hodgkin's disease
lupus erythematosis
scleroderma
arthritis
sarcoidosis
chronic respiratory disease
myasthenia gravis
autism
alcoholism
anorexia nervosa
bulimia
multiple sclerosis
drug addiction
inflammatory bowel disease

DRUGS THAT ENCOURAGE YEAST GROWTH

Antibiotics

amoxicillin
ampicillin
bactrim
ceclor
erythromicin
keflex
penicillin
septra
tetracycline
other antibiotics

Cortisone-type drugs

cortisone
decadron
prednisone

Oral contraceptives

Chemotherapeutic drugs

Any drug that is more stressful than helpful

Pregnancy—a factor in yeast overgrowth

Hormonal changes during pregnancy may encourage yeast overgrowth.

Food cravings that usually accompany yeast overgrowth

Sweets—This includes all forms of sugar: honey, white sugar, brown sugar, molasses, syrups and products containing any of these ingredients.

cheese
milk
ice cream
chocolate
peanut butter and/or
  peanuts
yeast bread
cereal grains—oatmeal,
  wheat, barley, rye,
  buckwheat, millet, rice
high carbohydrate foods
  such as potatoes and pasta

dried fruit
fruit juice
fresh fruit
vinegar and pickled foods
sauerkraut
smoked meats
smoked fish
soy sauce
alcoholic beverages,
  especially beer and wine
soft drinks
tea, including herb teas

SENSITIVITY TO MOLD
CAN BE RELATED TO CANDIDIASIS

If you do not feel as healthy as usual on rainy, damp days, you may be reacting to mold spores in the air. On damp days, airborne fungi multiply rapidly. People with candidiasis often have allergic reactions to other forms of fungi, such as those in the air.

Mold and fungi grow in dark, damp places—in bathrooms, under kitchen sinks, in basements, in cellars, in poorly ventilated closets and even in wallpaper and carpet. If you feel less than your best in certain areas of your home or office, maybe there is mold there. Your reaction can mean that your immune system, which in a healthy state could deal with common household fungi, is depressed by fungi growing within your body. Because of that depression of your immune system, you are now reacting to common household fungi and molds which normally would not bother you.

In diagnosing candidiasis, physicians usually investigate the possibility of mold allergies. The doctor may perform a laboratory test or simply quiz you to see if you have mold allergy symptoms. Mold allergy does not mean that you definitely have a Candida problem. Your doctor will make that determination based on a combination of factors.

VI RECOVERY: *The Back-to-Health Process*

DO YOU SUSPECT, after reading the signals of yeast overgrowth, that your health is being affected by Candida albicans? Has a physician, after carefully evaluating your health history and present condition, suggested that you have a yeast problem?

If your answer is "yes," the next step is to relax. Yeast overgrowth is reversible. You have an opportunity to rebuild your health, and develop a lifestyle of health techniques that will not only support the healing of your yeast disease, but also will support the healing of other diseases. Even better, continuing your new healthy way of life will prevent the development of other health problems.

For most people with candidiasis, healing is a gradual process. It does not happen overnight. Just as most diseases develop over a period of time, they often heal in the same way. This does not mean that your yeast problems cannot disappear in an instant. That is also possible. If they don't do a quick vanishing act, remember that gradual healing still gets you to the place you want to be.

There are many routes to health, many paths to the

top of the mountain. Some individuals have experienced the healing of candidiasis through prayer and meditation, with little attention to diet, exercise or the use of anti-yeast drugs. Others have relied on diet alone. For many, a combination of healthy practices—diet, exercise, appropriate anti-yeast drugs, nutritional supplements, a clean environment, prayer and meditation, and an attitude of self-appreciation works best.

DIET

Candida albicans prefers sweets and starches. It has little use for protein—eggs, poultry, seafood or meat. It doesn't particularly like fats—butter or oil. The all-American diet of chocolate chip cookies, milk shakes, sugary soft drinks, donuts, ice cream and pancakes and syrup provide the ideal nutrition for any ambitious yeast colony with intentions of expanding.

Health sophisticates feed their Candida dried fruit and nut mixes, honey, blackstrap molasses, the purest maple syrup, carob candies, and enormous quantities of grains. Fresh fruit, reputed to be a health food, contains enough sugar to upset body chemistry and stimulate yeast growth. Fruit juices, loaded with sugar *au naturel*, are great for yeasts. Studies have shown Candida albicans to be growing rapidly in freshly squeezed orange juice.

Candida overgrowth often creates a sensitivity to other yeasts and molds. Vinegar and pickled foods, smoked meats and fish, and the baker's yeast in bread can evoke symptoms. Even inhaling the yeast in a bakery can be a problem for the extremely sensitive person.

The following outline includes most foods that

can encourage yeast overgrowth and/or stress the human immune system. If Candida is a factor in your health problems these guidelines suggest foods you want to eliminate from your diet.

A. Eating refined sugar weakens the immune system and also feeds yeast organisms. Overeating starchy foods also seems to encourage yeast growth.

1. Do not eat sugar or sweets. This includes products made with honey, molasses and syrup, as well as sugar.

2. Do not eat large portions of wheat, oats, rye, barley, corn, rice, potatoes or millet. Some people may need to limit their intake of these foods to 1 tablespoon per meal.

3. Milk sugar can encourage Candida overgrowth. Avoid milk and milk products except butter.

B. Many people with Candida overgrowth develop sensitivities and allergies to other yeasts and molds, which trigger symptoms and weaken the immune system. Yeast, mold and fungus should be minimized in foods.

1. Yeast is used in food preparation and flavoring of:
Commercial breads, rolls, coffee cakes, pastries, leavened crackers.
Beer, wine and all alcoholic beverages.
Most commercial soups, barbecue potato chips and dry roasted nuts.
Vinegar and vinegar-containing foods such as pickles, sauerkraut, relishes, green olives and salad dressing. (Lemon juice with oil may be used as a yeast-free salad dressing.)

Soy sauce, tofu, miso, cider and natural root beer.

2. Yeast is the basis for many vitamin and mineral preparations; for instance, tryptophan is often derived from yeast.

3. Molds grow on foods while drying, soaking, curing and fermenting.

   Avoid pickled, smoked or dried meats, fish and poultry, including sausages, salami, hot dogs, pickled tongue, corned beef, pastrami, smoked sardines and other fish that have been dried or smoked.

   Bacon and country-style cured pork of all kinds is usually coated with mold.

   Dried fruits such as prunes, raisins, dates, figs, citrus peels, candied cherries, currants, peaches, apples and apricots should also be avoided.

   All cheeses including cottage cheese are moldy and should be avoided.

   Dried teas, including herb teas can be a source of mold.

4. Mold grows on all vegetables. Wash foods well before eating.

5. Avoid canned or frozen citrus, grape and tomato juice. Aside from containing too much natural sugar, citric acid is often added to these products. Citric acid is a by-product of yeast and may provoke reactions.

6. Mushrooms are a member of the fungi family. Some people with Candida overgrowth appear to be allergic to mushrooms.

7. Peanuts often support the growth of a toxic mold called aflatoxin. Avoid peanuts and peanut butter.

C. Eating fruit will boost blood sugar levels and encourage growth. Fruit and fruit juices must be omitted from the diet.

Just reading this list could be a test for Candida overgrowth. If you have candidiasis, you probably began hyperventilating half way through the list. By now you are breaking out in a sweat, your pulse is above normal, and a sense of panic is taking over. These are all your favorite foods.

Candida overgrowth brings a craving for most of these forbidden foods—not just a preference, but a strong, virtually insatiable craving. People report dragging themselves out of bed at 2:00 A.M. to go to the all-night grocery. The grocery list is simple: chocolate malt balls or peanut butter candy. Others find that, even though they know better, they eat ice cream for dinner. Often, one completely loses the desire for high quality protein and fresh vegetables. The refrigerator has no room for these items. It's brimming over with milk, cheeses, fruit, ice cream, peanut butter, soft drinks and beer.

The irony of this situation is apparent. It appears that one is autonomous—eating for his or her own benefit and pleasure, making independent decisions about what to put into the grocery cart—but is this really what is taking place? Maybe not. Maybe Candida's food preferences are now overriding healthy human ones. Maybe the yeast overgrowth has altered body chemistry in such a way that it is dictating the daily menu.

Candida often seems completely in control of the situation. Nutritionists who assist Candida patients in planning a healing diet see stubborn resistance to eliminating yeast foods. Some patients weep as they read the list of foods they must avoid. Sophisticated, mature women raise their voices: "You mean

I can't eat peanut butter sandwiches? My favorite food?" But most people then reach the stage of acceptance and ask what is left to eat?

Here's where the good news comes in. The following lists include foods that one can enjoy on a pro-human, anti-Candida diet! They are divided into seven major groups which form the basis of the Rainbow Meal Plan which we'll come to next.

ONE: *Complete Protein*

Meats

beef	gelatin, plain	mutton
beef brains	goat meat	rabbit
beef heart	goose	sweetbreads
beef tongue	kidney	veal
buffalo	lamb	wild
frog legs	liver	*squirrel, deer*

Fowl

chicken	organ meats	pheasant
duck	*from chicken,*	turkey
	turkey, etc.	

Eggs

chicken	duck	goose

Fish, Mollusks and Crustaceans

abalone	haddock	salmon
anchovy	halibut	sardine
bass	herring	scallop
carp	lobster	shark
caviar	mackerel	shrimp
clam	*Spanish*	smelt
cod	mullet	sole
crab	*Lisa*	sunfish
crappie	oysters	swordfish
crayfish	perch	tuna
fish roe	pompano	white fish
flounder	red snapper	whiting

TWO: *Grains and Legumes*

Grains

amaranth	millet	rice
barley	oats	*brown*
buckwheat	oat bran	sprouted grains
corn	psyllium seed	*barley, wheat,*
flaxseed	husks	rye

Legumes

beans	*peas*	lentils
azuki	black-eyed	
black	chick	
kidney	*garbanzos*	
lima	snap	
navy	split	
pinto		
soy		
string		
mung		

THREE: *Root Vegetables*

artichokes	onion	radish
Jerusalem	parsnip	rutabaga
anise root	parsley root	turnip
beet	Irish potato	yam
carrot	sweet potato	
celeriac		
celery root		
kohlrabi		

FOUR: *Yellow and white vegetables*

avocado	cucumber	rutabaga
bean sprouts, mung	endive, Belgian	squash
beans, wax	jicama	*yellow, crook-*
cauliflower	onion	*necked*
corn	parsnip	turnip
	radish	

FIVE: *Green vegetables*

artichoke, globe	celery	peas, green
asparagus	leeks	peas, sugar snap
bean, lima	okra	pepper, green
beans, string	olive	sprouts
broccoli	pea-pods	scallions
	edible	zucchini

SIX: *Red, orange and purple vegetables*

beets	red cabbage	winter squash
carrots	red bell peppers	yam
eggplant	sweet potato	
pumpkin	tomato	

SEVEN: *Leafy green vegetables*

artichokes	dandelion	parsley
beet tops	endive	spinach
bok choy	escarole	summer savory
brussels sprouts	kale	turnip greens
cabbage	lettuce, iceberg	watercress
chicory	lettuce, red leaf	Swiss chard
chives	lettuce, romaine	sunflower greens
collards	mustard greens	

As you can see, your starvation is not an issue. Starvation of Candida is the issue. These vegetables, proteins, whole grains, fresh herbs and condiments are not Candida's food preferences.

Clinical research spanning many decades has shown these foods to be the best for humans. Free of sugar and caffeine, they are not likely to be stressful.

Some individuals with Candida overgrowth have developed food allergies or sensitivities. Some of these can be glaringly obvious. Eating eggs results in an instant headache. Have a shrimp and break out in hives. Even good foods, such as eggs or shrimps, can be problem foods temporarily. If you suspect food allergies, keep a diet diary and observe the connection between what you have eaten and how you feel. A little detective work can usually isolate the foods you need to avoid for awhile.

By eating only small portions you can often minimize allergic reactions. An ideal meal plan with built-in small portions is the Rainbow Meal Plan. Here is the menu for a sample meal:

Leafy Green
Vegetable
Spinach

Red Vegetable
Tomato

Grain or Legume
Brown rice

Complete Protein
Beef

Root Vegetable
Potato

Yellow Vegetable
Squash

Green Vegetable
Asparagus

Notice that one food from each of the vegetable categories on the recommended food list is on the menu. There is a red, a green, a green leafy, a yellow and a root vegetable. Then there is a small serving of a whole grain or bean. A modest serving of a complete protein rounds out the meal. This is not an unusual way of eating. The traditional American meal—tossed salad, baked potato, steamed broccoli, and steak, chicken or seafood—is a Rainbow Meal.

The only difference here is in the size of the portions. When we eat large portions, sometimes digestion is not complete. Undigested food becomes toxic as it passes through the intestines. The toxins that are released can cause health problems and prevent healing. Small portions allow more complete digestion. There is also less chance of an allergic reaction.

Most people can eat portions of about one-fourth cup. With seven items in a meal, that totals almost two cups of food. Some people may need to eat only three of these meals daily. Others may find four or five mini-meals to be ideal.

An extremely ill person will want to eat only one tablespoon of each food. Since seven items are on the plate, this totals about one half cup of food. Not much, right? That means that this person will need to eat frequently, maybe every two hours during the day.

Eat every two hours! Who wants to be a slave to the stove? These meals do not require kitchen bondage. Half of the meal can be eaten raw, as a salad. Steaming is the ideal way to cook the remainder of the food. Even the protein is delicious when steamed. Stainless steel steamers can be purchased in most grocery store gadget sections. These flowerette designed utensils fit into almost any size saucepan. As water boils in the bottom of the saucepan, the steam rises through the little holes in the steamer basket, gently cooking the slices of vegetables and small portions of protein. Moisture is retained and added to the foods. Vitamins are not destroyed by excessive and prolonged heat. A meal can be ready, from refrigerator to table, in less than 10 minutes.

Another wonderful way to cook a Rainbow Meal

is in a crock pot. These slow cookers do not over-heat foods. Even with no imagination, you can pro-duce savory soups and stews. Start with good-quality pure water, then simply add equal portions of each of the seven categories of foods. The slow, even simmering of the crock pot will gently blend the flavors in a way that is fail proof. These soups and stews can be taken to work in a thermos, frozen for later eating or kept in the refrigerator, to be ready for instant eating.

In some cases, varying your foods so that the same items are not eaten day after day is helpful. If you wish to rotate your diet on a four-day plan, use the list that follows to make planning easy.

Four-Day Rotation Diet*

DAY ONE	DAY TWO

Protein:

Egg	Beef
Lamb	Liver, calves
Veal	Anchovy
Crab	Flounder
Herring	Lobster
Mussels	Oyster
Red snapper	Salmon
Sea bass	Shrimp
	Tuna

Leafy Green Vegetables:

Artichoke	Brussels sprouts
Collard greens	Endive
Parsley	Romaine lettuce

Green Vegetables:

Asparagus	Broccoli
Leeks	Okra
Sprouts, mung bean	

Yellow/White Vegetables:

Avocado	Cauliflower
Squash, acorn	Squash, yellow

Red/Orange/Purple/ Vegetables:

Beets	Carrots
	Tomato

Root Vegetables:

Kohlrabi	Onions
	Rutabaga

Grains, Legumes & Beans:

Beans, azuki	Beans, black
Beans, navy	Beans, pinto
Lentil	Millet
Peas, green	Rice, brown
Buckwheat	Oats

DAY THREE

Chicken
Pork
Clam
Grouper
Mackerel
Perch
Sardine
Sole
Trout

Cabbage
Iceberg lettuce
Spinach

Celery
Scallions

Corn
Squash, zucchini

Eggplant
Sweet potato

Parsnips
Turnips (bottom)

Bean, kidney
Bean, soy
Pea, black-eyed
Rice, wild
Rye

DAY FOUR

Duck
Turkey
Cod
Halibut
Mullet
Pompano
Scallops
Swordfish

Chives
Mustard greens
Swiss chard
Watercress

Green pepper
Sprouts, alfalfa

Cucumber
Yellow wax beans

Pumpkin

Potato, white
Radish

Bean, lima
Bean, string
Pea, chick
Barley
Wheat

*This diet provided by Physicians Cyto Laboratories, Fort Lauderdale, Florida

How about eating out? Is it possible to find a Rainbow Meal in a restaurant? Not only possible, easy! Most restaurants are sporting salad bars. Add a baked potato. You don't have to eat the entire giant spud. Learn to disobey the compulsion to clean all plates that are put before you. Add a small portion of seafood, meat, poultry or an egg, and you have your little rainbow.

Assert yourself politely with restaurant personnel. It's their business to please you. If you want your protein cooked without any sugar or chemical-laden sauces, ask for it that way. Even though the menu boasts chicken poached in wine sauce, the chef will usually be glad to cook yours in a more simple manner.

If you dine with a friend, share an entree. Restaurants usually serve enough protein on one plate for two or three people. Each of you can order a salad or go to the salad bar, then you can share a potato and the protein. You will leave with more money in your wallet and less discomfort in your abdomen.

Many people find these Rainbow Meals to be a satisfying way of eating. The meals are beautiful, the bright vegetable colors contrasting with earthy beans and whole grains. Variety is indeed one of the spices of life, and these meals guarantee variety in color, texture, tastes, vitamins, minerals and enzymes. Discovering the tastes of new foods can be delightful. If you have been in a dietary rut, eating your four favorite foods repeatedly, this plan will allow you to escape that rut.

Some people find the Rainbow Meals too structured, too disciplined. They resent counting to seven and buying so many different items. If this is so, choose what is called a Modified Food Plan. This meal plan simply eliminates foods that encourage Candida growth and combines protein with carbohydrates and fats for a balanced meal. The number of different foods on the plate may be only two or three instead of seven. An example of a meal from the Modified Food Plan would be fish and potato, lettuce and tomato salad.

Many people prefer to eat some meals from the Rainbow Plan and some from the Modified Food Plan. Breakfast of oat bran cereal, butter and a soft boiled egg would be from the Modified Food Plan. Lunch of homemade soup could be a compact Rainbow Meal. Dinner of tossed salad, brown rice and fish could qualify as Rainbow or Modified, depending on the number of different items included.

Either of these eating plans is excellent. A combination of the two plans seems to offer the most variety, ease of preparation and planning.

Let eating be a part of your life that is easy, effortless and stress-free. If you become compulsive, obsessed with planning your meals, refusing to eat in restaurants, resentful of a special diet, don't expect health to be around the next corner. Consider seeing this way of eating as an opportunity to love yourself. Make it pleasant. Begin each meal with a sense of gratitude. Instead of nourishing Candida, you are nourishing you!

Here are tips for shopping.

ANTI-CANDIDA SHOPPING

For the yeast-free special diet or the yeast-free low-carbohydrate diet plans, supermarket shopping is easier than ever before. In general, you can bypass about 80 percent of the foods offered, and head directly to a few sections:

MEATS Select fresh lean meats, poultry and fish. Avoid ground meat, pork, breaded and pickled meats, or any processed meat with additives. Some frozen food can be stored for convenience—for instance, keep a bag of frozen (unbreaded) scallops on hand—it's so easy to thaw a few for a quick meal, and reseal the package.

DAIRY PRODUCTS Select fresh eggs and unsalted butter and ignore the rest. Look for the date on the egg cartons.

SEEDS, NUTS AND GRAINS These may be found in bulk packages. Be sure to use brown rice and whole grains.

PRODUCE Pass up the fruit section. Select vegetables that look fresh and free of mold.

CONDIMENTS Select olive oil, spices, herbs and sea salt.

CANNED GOODS A few canned goods (without additives), such as tomato paste, water chestnuts, olives, tuna and sardines are acceptable for emergencies. Choose canned tomato products without citric acid.

FROZEN VEGETABLES Stock some such as frozen artichoke hearts or green peas for soups and salads. Check labels and avoid those with sugar, vinegar and additives.

DELI SECTION Select corn tortillas and shun everything else. Check the label carefully to avoid preservatives.

CRACKERS If you can't find yeast- and sugar-free wholegrain crackers in the supermarket, look for them in the health food store.

CAUTION Don't overbuy! Purchase fresh foods

frequently, as soon as possible after they are delivered to the store.*

From the *Candida Albicans Yeast-Free Cookbook*, here are more simple guidelines:

1. Prepare and eat small portions (these may range from an eighth to a quarter of a cup in the beginning).
2. For a Rainbow Meal, choose one food from each category.
3. All vegetables should be raw or gently steamed, not overcooked.
4. Kelp powder, sea salt, plain pepper and raw butter can be used in moderation.
5. Digestion begins in your mouth. Chew thoroughly and enjoy every bite.
6. Drink only distilled water. Sip small amounts with meals and drink at least eight glasses a day between meals.
7. Eat as many meals per day as desired. Use these meals for a snack; conform to these guidelines and space your meals at least two hours apart.
8. To aid digestion, relax before, during and after your meals. Keep your thoughts and conversation calm.

*These suggestions are reprinted from *The Candida Albicans Yeast-Free Cookbook*, by Pat Connolly. (Keats Publishing, Inc. New Canaan, Connecticut, 1985). If you want to recover completely from candidiasis, you want Pat Connolly's book in your kitchen. It offers delicious, easy, original recipes and is chock-full of tips that can make the difference in rebuilding your health.

ANTI-YEAST MEDICATIONS AND THERAPIES

It is possible to reverse Candida overgrowth without the use of anti-yeast drugs. In most cases, however, appropriate use of anti-yeast medication gives the body the boost it needs to gain the upper hand in controlling Candida. There are several medications that have been used with great success. These prescription drugs have few, if any side effects.

The most widely used medication is nystatin, named for the New York state laboratory where it was developed over thirty years ago. Since that time, it has been used to treat adults, children and even infants. The *Physicians' Desk Reference* describes nystatin as "virtually nontoxic and nonsensitizing and is well tolerated by all groups, even on prolonged administration." Of all the drugs available, nystatin is known for its effectiveness and safety.

It seems that nystatin kills yeast cells on contact. When it is swallowed, most of the drug remains in the digestive tract where it does its work. Little or none is absorbed into the bloodstream. Tablets, powder and liquid nystatin are made for oral use.

What about vaginal yeast infections? Suppositories of nystatin are effective here. For yeast overgrowth on skin and nails, ointments, powder and creams are available.

Many physicians have found that some of the commercial nystatin products are limited in their effectiveness. The suppositories made by pharmaceutical companies are in a base of lactose, milk sugar, which itself can be a food for yeast. The liquid suspension is often in a base of 50 percent sucrose: that's sugar, yeast's favorite item on any menu. Patients with allergies and sensitivities may respond poorly to the dyes and preservatives used in these commercial products. To avoid questionable ingredients, many physicians prescribe pure nystatin powder.

The best dose of nystatin powder is usually determined by trial and error. Frequently the starting dose is ¹⁄₁₆ to ⅛ teaspoon, four times daily. It can be stirred into a little water, swished around in the mouth before swallowing, and it will do its job of killing yeast cells from mouth to rectum. Some patients prefer to put the powder on their tongue and let it gradually mix with the saliva, then swallow it slowly. Its slightly bitter taste is not offensive.

Other patients prefer to mix one day's complete dose in eight ounces of water, carrying it with them in a plastic bottle, and sipping it often throughout the day.

Some people complain that mixing the powder is inconvenient when traveling or working. They prefer the commercially prepared tablets. One tablet is equivalent to ⅛th teaspoon of powder. Tablets can be broken up for smaller doses.

Homemade vaginal suppositories can be prepared by purchasing clear gelatin capsules in a health food store or pharmacy and filling them with the powder. A number two gelatin capsule holds ⅛th teaspoon or 500,000 units of nystatin powder. To prepare a suppository, place a small amount of powder on a clean piece of paper and fill without tightly packing the capsule. A vaginal applicator can be purchased at a pharmacy. Moisten the capsule so that it will adhere to the applicator without falling out before it can be inserted. Insertion into the vagina before bed will allow nystatin to kill neighborhood yeasts during the night.

Inventive patients have found many ways to use nystatin. One mixed the powder with distilled water and put the drug into her ears. The chronic ear trouble she had experienced for years began to clear immediately.

Another determined woman developed nystatin colon implants, very effective at killing yeast in the lower bowel. Here's her protocol for clearing Candida from the large intestine. Before bed, flush the bowel clean with a plain tepid water enema. After all the liquid has been expelled, mix approximately one-half teaspoon of nystatin powder with one cup of tepid water. Pour this mixture into an enema bag or enema bucket, let it run into the colon, and retain the fluid. Go directly to bed. This small amount of fluid will not give the urge to evacuate. Nystatin powder gains direct exposure to the yeast in the lower bowel and can work very efficiently.

A similar implant into the vaginal vault is very potent in killing yeast colonies that affect female sex organs. Mix one-half teaspoon nystatin powder with eight ounces of pure water. Put this into a douche bag and, lying down, let the fluid run into the vaginal canal. Remain in a reclining position, retaining this mixture for at least ten minutes. Stand in a tub or shower and let it drain effortlessly. For convenience, this entire procedure can be done lying in a tub. For comfort, lie on a towel or in a little hot water.

Sniffing the yellow nystatin powder is reported to be helpful in relieving sinus symptoms. Street talk is helpful in giving these directions. While pressing closed one nostril, snort powder from the tip of your finger into the other nostril. Some patients have elegant nystatin sniffers, purchased at "head shops." A less dramatic way of getting nystatin into areas of nasal congestion is simply to shake your container of powder vigorously, then remove the lid and hold the container under your nose. Sniff or inhale gently. Many people find that this technique clears not only nasal congestion, but also clears mental fuzziness and feelings of nervousness.

Although most patients do well on nystatin, some have unpleasant reactions. Headaches, fatigue, ache-all-over sensations and flu-like symptoms, including fever may develop during the first few days of treatment. Often this means that the dose is too large. It is thought that these reactions are partially due to the die off of yeast, and the resulting toxins which the body is unable to process quickly enough to avoid unpleasant reactions.

Some patients find that they do best when they take only a "dot" dose of nystatin powder. This is the amount that you can gather on the end of a flat toothpick, then put into your mouth. These people often begin with one dot dose every two days. If that produces no uncomfortable side effects, they increase the frequency and size of the dose until they see definite improvement.

Although some individuals cannot tolerate nystatin, even in small doses, it is by far the safest and most uniformly effective of all the anti-yeast medications. Nystatin tablets are marketed by Squibb under the name Mycostatin and by Lederle under the brand name Nilstat. Generic tablets, oral suspensions, vaginal suppositories and powders for topical use are also available. The pure nystatin powder is made by the American Cyanamid Company, Lederle Division. Physicians, hospitals, clinics and pharmacies can call 1-800-LEDERLE for more information.

For individuals who do not respond well to nystatin, there are other anti-yeast medications. One of these is ketoconazole, sold under the name Nizoral. Janssen Pharmaceutica developed this drug over a twenty-year period of research. It has been studied in nineteen countries in over 1,600 patients and has produced impressive results.

Nizoral has one clear advantage over nystatin. It is absorbed into the bloodstream. As the blood transports it to various tissues, it can kill yeast colonies wherever they are flourishing: in the kidneys, lungs, brain or vagina. Since Nizoral affects the system of the entire body, it is called a systemic drug. This is unlike nystatin, whose activity is mainly limited to the digestive tract or just the area where it is inhaled, inserted, implanted or applied.

The University of Texas Health Center in San Antonio has done research using Nizoral to treat oral thrush, candidiasis in the mouth. Doctors reported a 74 percent cure. In children up to two and one-half years old, over 90 percent responded. Similar studies with vaginal candidiasis—itching, discharge, inflammation—looked good. One tablet daily for six days brought relief for 80 percent of these women.

Chronic fungus infections of the skin can clear rapidly with Nizoral. Emory University worked with patients whose skin infections had persisted for an average of twenty years. Out of twenty such stubborn cases, infections cleared completely in thirteen people. All patients experienced 90 percent improvement. Progress was rapid. Within a week after beginning the drug, results were obvious.

One of these Emory patients was a man whose fungus infection has lasted for twenty-five years. On the 90 percent of his body that the infection covered, he experienced itching and scaling of his skin. After only five days on Nizoral, these symptoms began to diminish. After fifty-six days of drug therapy, his skin was totally clear. It is no surprise that the chairman of Emory's dermatology department says that this drug "heralds the beginning of a new era."

With such accolades to its credit, why isn't Nizoral

always chosen over nystatin? Unlike nystatin, whose side effects are usually minor, Nizoral can occasionally cause liver inflammation. The manufacturer's label is required to carry this warning: "It's important to perform liver function tests . . . before treatment and at periodic intervals during treatment (monthly or more frequently), particularly in patients who will be on prolonged therapy or have a history of liver disease." Reported cases of liver inflammation are rare. Many physicians find that Nizoral is more effective than nystatin in dealing with colonies of yeast that are well-established outside the digestive tract.

Clotrimazole is a drug that is sold in the form of a cream, ointment and suppositories. The cream and ointment are effective in treating skin infections. But since the suppositories are formulated in a lactose base, and lactose is thought to feed Candida, the suppositories are not considered suitable treatment.

Like nystatin, oral Amphotericin B is not absorbed out of the intestinal tract. It is also known to be effective at treating candidiasis and is relatively nontoxic. France is the place to get it; at this time, it is manufactured in this country only in a pill combined with tetracycline. Remember, tetracycline is one of Candida's favorite meals. The tetracycline-free Amphotericin B capsules are marketed in France under the name Fungizone.

There are many other drugs, both prescription and over-the-counter, that are being used topically and internally to assist the body's immune system in overcoming yeast infections. If you have a yeast problem, a physician experienced in dealing with candidiasis and other fungus infections can help determine which, if any, is best for you.

Yeast vaccines have been helpful in many cases

of candidiasis. Vaccine stimulates the body's white blood cells to deal more vigorously and efficiently with Candida. This is the same principle as the vaccines given to protect against tetanus, whooping cough and polio.

However, there are some problems with Candida vaccines. There are many different strains of Candida yeast. The yeast from which the vaccine was made may not be the strain of yeast in the patient to whom it is given. Determining the proper dose can also be a dilemma. A dose that works one day may not be ideal on another day. Obviously, the use of yeast vaccine requires an experienced physician who is willing to monitor carefully the patient's response.

Homeopathy is a medical specialty originating in nineteenth century Germany. The principle is "like cures like." A homeopathic physician administers minute dilutions of the substance thought to be the cause of the ailment. These pills or drops seem to stimulate the body to respond in a way that eliminates the problem. There is little documentation for homeopathy, few articles in scientific journals. There are many anecdotes and devoted practitioners who report impressive results. Homeopathic remedies for Candida albicans overgrowth are available and most homeopathic physicians are also licensed medical doctors.

Long before the advent of modern drugs, homeopathic remedies and plants were used to stimulate cures. Medicinal plants came to be called herbs; their roots, leaves, bark and flowers were used to prepare medications.

Many candidiasis patients have claimed health benefits from an herb tea brewed from the inner bark of a South American tree. This tree, *Tabebuia altissima*, grows in the Andes and has been medicinally used by the Indians for centuries. Two contemporary Argentinian physicians recently introduced the herb to the outside world. They claim that it has antibiotic capabilities without the side effects of our modern antibiotic drugs.

Taheebo is the Indian name for this herb and the tea is often marketed under this name. Other names include *Ipe Roxo*, Portuguese, or *Lapacho* or *Tabebuia*, Spanish names. It is also called Pau d'Arco.

When this tea is combined with a culture of Candida albicans in a laboratory there is no yeast die-off, which may mean that taheebo is of no use in healing candidiasis or perhaps it simply means that the activity of taheebo is somehow mediated through the body. Possibly, taheebo stimulates immune mechanisms to defeat Candida.

While some patients report dramatic results with this remedy, others see no effects. Trial and error or trial and success seem to be the best method to see if it is of value.

Here is Pat Connolly's recipe from the *Candida Albicans Yeast-Free Cookbook*:

TAHEEBO OR PAU D'ARCO TEA

It is brewed as follows:

1 heaping tablespoon tea or the contents of 3 tea bags emptied into pot
1 quart water

Add the water to the tea and simmer on the lowest heat possible for at least half an hour. Allow the liquid to cool and pour into a storage jar with a tight-fitting lid. Refrigerate. Sip the chilled tea as desired. Adjust the recipe to make enough to be completely consumed in two days.

During the initial days or weeks of anti-Candida therapy, one may feel worse. Aches and pains may intensify, fatigue may become more severe, sore throats and flu-like symptoms may blossom. Scientists say that this is the result of toxins released by dead or dying organisms—in this case, Candida albicans.

This reaction is common when one begins therapy with a large dose of any of the anti-yeast drugs or natural remedies. The reaction is called the Herxheimer reaction. It can often be avoided by beginning treatment with dietary changes first. After a week or two on an anti-Candida diet as outlined in this book, begin prescription or non-prescription remedies at a low dosage. If the small amount is well tolerated, increase gradually to a full dosage. This protocol keeps yeast die-off at a moderate rate and gives the body time to handle the toxins and efficiently dispose of dead and dying yeast.

NUTRITIONAL THERAPY FOR YEAST OVER-GROWTH

Vitamins, minerals, amino acids and essential fatty acids are necessary for your vitality. Without them, life does not go on. In an age of depleted top-soil, prolonged food storage, artificially induced ripeness and overcooking, most foods do not supply the nutritional components needed to make bodies work well. Breakdowns result. Candidiasis is one of those breakdowns.

Which came first, the chicken or the egg? Which came first, candidiasis or nutrient deficiencies? Nutrient deficiencies can certainly set the stage for yeast overgrowth by weakening the immune system and creating a need for antibiotic treatment for persistent infections. Once Candida is cozily nestled into the tissues, its toxins are stressful, depleting the body of nutrients, creating deficiencies.

Most health professionals have observed that patients with chronic yeast problems appear to have nutritional deficiencies also. Along with anti-yeast medication and a healing, nutrient-rich diet, most physicians recommend a supplementation program of vitamins and minerals. Some may also add digestive enzymes, amino acids, and special supplements they have found to be helpful.

Vitamin A works to protect from infection the mucous membranes of the mouth, throat, intestines, vagina, urinary tract and lungs. Without enough of this nutrient, the special cells in these areas do not produce the lubricating mucus needed for defense. Instead they become hard and defenseless against infection. Since these mucous membranes are the most common sites of Candida infection, it makes sense to get adequate vitamin A into the diet. Animal studies have shown that there is less susceptibility to candidiasis when vitamin A is supplied in high doses.

Liver is a rich food source of this nutrient. A three-ounce serving provides about 45,000 IU. Color gives the clue to vitamin A content in vegetables. A dark orange carrot has lots more vitamin A than a pale yellow one. Dark green vegetables are a good source as are bright yellow ones. Deep rich hues say, "Vitamin A found here." Food supplements of vitamin A are commonly prescribed. Although there are many rumors of vitamin A toxicity, this is a phenomenon rarely seen.

B vitamins are so busy that they would require their own book to be described adequately. They are really a family of vitamins: B1, B2, B3, B5, B6, B12 and other cousins. The B-complex family is in the business of energy production, maintenance of the nervous system and proper handling of fats, proteins and carbohydrates. They are also specialists in continuous remodeling and renovation of the skin, hair, eyes, mouth and liver.

These heroes of human life are destroyed by sugar and alcohol. They are depleted by coffee and excessive carbohydrates. Food processors extract them from most of their products.

Do you know any Americans who are tired, irritable, nervous or depressed? Those are classic symptoms of B-vitamin deficiencies. Add a little grey hair, hair loss, insomnia and constipation and you have a textbook description of the need for more B vitamins.

Many B-complex vitamin supplements are made with a yeast base. Candidiasis often creates an allergy to this yeast base, so read vitamin labels carefully to find yeast-free ones. If you appear to have a severe vitamin B deficiency, your physician may advise injections as well as oral supplementation of this important group of nutrients.

Your physician may want to take a special look at the possibility of a vitamin B6 deficiency, which may require extra B6 supplementation in addition to the B-complex supplement. Vitamin B6 deficiency is thought to be very common. This is a nutrient you don't want to be without.

B6 plays a leading role in many important human chemical dramas. It gets protein molecules together. It transfers molecules from one location to another. It helps unite chemicals that would not socialize without it. Red blood cells depend on it for growth and normal function. Fat and carbohydrate metabolism will not work properly without B6. That also holds true for the metabolism of fatty acids and cholesterol.

B6 deficiency could easily play a role in the food

cravings experienced by many candidiasis patients. Adequate B6 is necessary to convert stored muscle sugar (glycogen) into blood sugar (glucose) for a steady energy supply. When blood sugar drops without enough B6 to change muscle sugar quickly, the brain needs a snack to get the blood sugar back up. The snack that gets the blood sugar up fast is sugar. Any other carbohydrate will also work: rice cakes, bread, potatoes, fruit.

Mood-elevating brain chemicals could also be a factor in food cravings linked with candidiasis. B6 and tryptophan, an amino acid, work together to form serotonin, a neurotransmitter that prevents depression. Without enough B6 or with low amino acid levels, this peace and contentment brain chemical doesn't get made. High fat diets make tryptophan more available to the brain. High sucrose content in the diet has also been found to lead to increased serotonin brain levels. Maybe this is the reason that peanut butter sandwiches, dried fruit and nut mixes, butter and rice cakes or ice cream readily come to the minds of most Candida comrades.

B6 is a vitamin that is not always used efficiently in a person with metabolic problems. To insure that you actually benefit from the supplement you take, your physician may choose to prescribe a form of this vitamin called pyridoxal-5-phosphate.

Vitamin C (ascorbic acid) has been the called "the healing factor." Its role in human health is awesomely varied. An essential ingredient in the formation of collagen, the protein that forms skin, ligaments, bones and other connective tissue, vitamin C literally keeps us together. Since tissue strength is critically important in preventing Candida overgrowth, vitamin C is vital to a supplement program. Additional benefits include its ability to reduce the affects of allergens and quell allergic reactions typical of candidiasis patients. This nutrient will also assist completion of many of the body's chemical reactions. It is thought to play a role in calcium metabolism, and protects many other nutrients from destruction by oxidation.

Like all supplement recommendations, that for vitamin C is an individual affair. It is readily available in tablet or powder form. The powder, or crystals dissolve conveniently in water and may be sipped throughout the day. Extremely sensitive individuals may want to use a highly purified hypoallergenic form of this vitamin, usually derived from Sago palm rather than corn. Intravenous vitamin C has been used with great success in the treatment of candidiasis and other immune system disorders. A four-hour intravenous drip may contain up to 60,000 milligrams of ascorbic acid.

Robert S. London, M.D. reported in the *Journal of the American College of Nutrition* (2:115–122, 1983) that vitamin E supplementation provided relief from nervous tension, mood swings, craving for sweets, fatigue, forgetfulness, increased appetite and depression—all common symptoms of Candida overgrowth. The optimal dose seemed to be 300 IU daily.

Minerals are another important group of chemicals that sustain our lives. They make up 4 percent of our total weight. Calcium, chloride, chromium, cobalt, copper, fluoride, iodine, iron, magnesium, manganese, molybdenum, phosphorus, potassium, selenium, sodium, sulfur and zinc are all necessary for optimum health. When designing a supplement program, experienced nutritional physicians usually correlate blood chemistry, hair analysis, urinalysis and health history and symptoms. By studying lab results and getting to know the health problems of the patient, the physician can prescribe personalized mineral supplementation.

It is important to remember that eating sugar prevents minerals from functioning. The greatest mineral supplement made cannot withstand the onslaught of a sugar binge. This was scientifically researched by the late Dr. Melvin Page who found that sugar wrecks mineral relationships in the body. It somehow changes electrical charges making minerals react abnormally.

Do not be deceived into believing that vitamin and mineral supplements can make up for an abusive diet. Diet is the chemical foundation and framework of a health-building program. Supplements may play a necessary role, but they will not compensate for frequent meals of ice cream sundaes or chocolate eclairs.

Most people find that as they continue to take food supplements, their food preferences change. They may lose the craving for sweets, or need to eat less frequently. As body chemistry begins to work more efficiently, hunger adjusts accordingly. Weight loss or gain in the desired direction becomes effortless. Energy can be maintained throughout the day.

To assist the immune system to overcome Candida, specific immune system boosters can make a difference. The thymus gland (described in chapter four), is the one that produces lymphocytes, specialized thymic blood cells which are the officers of the body's defense forces. Called T-cells, they are thought to control other blood cells by destroying bacteria and killing foreign antigens in the blood. These foreign antigens are often products of Candida albicans. *In vivo* studies made by A. Goldstein, M.D. suggest that thymus supplementation can be effective in increasing the number of T-lymphocytes in individuals with deficient levels. These supplements are available from Ecological Formulas, Concord, California.

Essential fatty acids are also needed for your immune system to function well. These chemicals, found in unprocessed oils, are used by the body to make a group of hormone-like substances called prostaglandins. Two excellent sources of essential fatty acids are evening primrose oil, available in capsule form, and linseed oil. Linseed oil can be purchased in health food stores and should be refrigerated once opened. It can be used with lemon juice as a salad dressing.

Restoration of colon health is of foremost importance in the control of Candida albicans. Over 400 species of microorganisms coexist in the human intestinal tract. In the healthy colon, they are in balance, none dominating. Antibiotic drugs and other drugs, as well as a high carbohydrate diet, can upset this balance and encourage Candida to flourish. Once Candida overgrows in the intestines, cravings for sweets seem to increase. As the diet shifts toward concentrated sugars and away from fresh vegetables, whole grains and complete proteins, further colon deterioration occurs.

Oral supplementation with *lactobacillus acidophilus* may help to reinoculate the bowel with favorable bacteria. Contrary to what you may think, commercial yogurt is not a good source of *lactobacillus acidophilus*. To insure active, live cultures of this friendly bacteria, consult your physician or health food store for a high-quality acidophilus supplement. It comes in capsules, powder and liquid form.

Liquid chlorophyll, known for its detoxifying properties, is rich in vitamin A and works to heal the mucous membranes that line the colon. Bentonite is another colon restorer. A tablespoon of colloidal bentonite may be taken before bed. Bentonite has strong adsorptive properties and can remove toxins from the colon; it can also remove valuable nutrients, so it is best taken hours after the last meal of the day and not at the same time as food supplements.

Herbal combinations of cascara sagrada bark, buckthorn bark, licorice root, capsicum fruit, ginger root, barberry root bark, couchgrass herb, red clover tops and lobelia can also be helpful in restoring colon health.

Lack of peristalsis, the rhythmic, wavelike contractions of the intestines, results in unhealthy changes in intestinal flora and in constipation. Both can be reversed by adding more fiber to the diet. Oat bran cereal is a rich source of high-quality fiber. For those not sensitive to oats, wheat or eggs, here's a high-fiber, colon-cleansing, easy breakfast that is also delicious:

> Into one cup of pure water stir one-quarter cup of oat bran cereal and one heaping tablespoon of wheat bran. Stir until lumps dissolve. Continue to stir and heat until simmering. Cook for one minute. Break a raw egg into the cereal and continue to stir gently so that the white cooks slightly. Pour into a bowl and add butter and salt if desired.

Oat bran contains a special fiber called beta-glucans. As beta-glucans travels through the intestines, it forms fatty acids. These fatty acids are thought to help regulate blood sugar levels and normalize cholesterol production by the liver. Fatty acids have also been found to be fungicidal, which means that they help to kill Candida albicans. Caprylic acid is reported to be especially effective against Candida and is available in supplement form under the name of Caprystatin.

Medical literature since the time of Hippocrates

has cited garlic's medicinal qualities. Research studies show that garlic is antifungal. Several reports claim that its potency in combating Candida albicans is equal or sometimes superior to the leading drugs. Garlic supplements may be easily obtained or you can make your own garlic concentrate. Pat Connolly has this to say about garlic in her *Candida Albicans Yeast-Free Cookbook*:

> Garlic is said to be antifungal. Many people suffering from Candida feel better when using more garlic than the ordinary amount used as a spicy seasoning. The simple way to extract garlic oil for concentrated use is with alcohol such as vodka.

> **Ingredients:**
> ½ pound peeled garlic
>   cloves
> 1 bottle (fifth or quart)
>   vodka or gin

Place the garlic cloves in the blender with 1 cup of alcohol. Blend the mixture until it becomes mush. Add a second cup of alcohol and blend. Pour into a quart jar. Rinse the blender with ⅓ cup of alcohol and add this to the jar. Cap the jar with a firm-sealing lid that cannot leak. Shake the jar daily just long enough to mix well. Repeat this procedure for 10 days. Each day thereafter check the jar for about 1 inch of garlic oil rising to the top. Remove the oil by gently skimming or pouring. Don't use any of the mash sediment.

Collect the oil in an eye-dropper bottle and use as seasoning or external remedy. It is delicious blended into softened butter to top vegetables or in the salad dressing. Each time oil is removed, add a little alcohol to the jar. When no more oil rises, discard the mush and make a new batch.

Your physician may suggest other supplements that have been found to be effective in controlling Candida: olive oil, biotin, amino acids. Current research and publications on candidiasis are voluminous. New recommendations for nutritional therapy are a valuable offshoot of that research. An experienced, well informed, nutritionally oriented doctor will share the latest information with you.

AVOID DRUGS THAT STIMULATE YEAST GROWTH

When they appeared on the scene, antibiotics were hailed as miracle drugs. Does that mean that these drugs are best used only when miracles are required—in life-threatening situations? Candida is raising this question. Feeding directly on many antibiotics and their by-products, Candida thrives on antibiotic therapy.

The irony is that antibiotics may be frequently prescribed for conditions which are, at least in part, caused by Candida overgrowth. An immune system weakened by Candida toxins is more susceptible to infections, which often prompt physicians to get out their prescription pads. That prescribed antibiotic further stimulates yeast overgrowth. The proverbial vicious cycle is at work.

Even more absurd, antibiotics are often prescribed for conditions for which they are ineffective. How many times has your physician prescribed an antibiotic for your sore throat or cough without taking a culture to identify the organism causing the problem? Most people have had many antibiotics and no cultures. Since 80 to 90 percent of these respiratory infections are a result of virus infections, not bacterial ones, they can't be helped by antibiotics. Antibiotics don't kill viruses.

If you have a sore throat, fever or cough, you can make it easier for your physician to help you by not demanding a prescription for antibiotic drugs. You can patiently wait for a culture to be done and accept the extra cost of the lab work.

When antibiotic therapy is necessary, avoid eating foods that are stressful—mainly sweets. Ignore foods that feed yeast until you have completed the drug therapy and your condition is healed. Your physician may prescribe nystatin or another antiyeast medication to be taken along with the antibiotic.

Birth control pills appeared shortly after broadspectrum antibiotics. Add the increased consumption of sugary processed foods and now we have the ingredients for a Candida calamity.

It is estimated that 35 percent of women on the Pill have chronic, severe yeast vaginitis. The progesterone content of the Pill seems to create the perfect vaginal environment for Candida to multiply.

There are many birth control alternatives. Avoiding the birth control pill is required if a woman wants to recover from chronic candidiasis.

Immunosupressant drugs do exactly what the name says. They suppress the immune system. How can one's immune system gain the strength to control Candida if it is being simultaneously suppressed by drugs? This won't work! If you are taking immunosuppressant drugs, maybe you are not getting to the source of your health problems. These drugs usually cover up symptoms and don't lead to healing.

Candida overgrowth can be a source of the symptoms for which these drugs are often prescribed.

Inflammatory conditions such as joint pains and swelling may be a response to Candida toxins. If so, temporarily relieving the pain or swelling with immunosuppressant drugs doesn't remove the cause. Why not make control of Candida the first step in dealing with inflammatory or autoimmune conditions?

Re-evaluation of any drug is helpful in allowing your body to recover from candidiasis. Re-evaluation of antibiotics, the Pill and immunosuppressants is mandatory.

DEALING WITH GLANDULAR IMBALANCES, TOXIC METALS AND POOR CIRCULATION

Any of the above factors can encourage Candida overgrowth. That overgrowth can further contribute to glandular problems, limit the body's ability to excrete metals, and adversely affect circulation.

How do you know if you have glandular imbalances? This analysis is a project for a physician. It may not be necessary for you to see an endocrinologist. If your physician has experience at evaluating the glandular system and is familiar with therapy for reestablishing balance, you may need to look no further.

Blood and urine testing will give your physician valuable information with which to make a diagnosis. Your symptoms, a physical examination, your health history and the health record of your parents will also be part of the diagnostic process.

The Page endocrine analysis developed by Dr. Melvin E. Page, is an accurate, economical and quick method of determining your genetic glandular potential. This technique reveals which glands are genetically overactive, underactive or perfectly normal. If you were born with an underactive thyroid gland and you have been chronically ill or experiencing significant stress, your thyroid gland will most likely have become even weaker—more underactive. If you were born with an overactive thyroid gland, stress will push it towards more overactivity.

The Page technique involves measuring the size of the legs at specific points below the knee and the size of the forearm at specific points. A mathematical computation is then plotted on a graph which reveals your genetic glandular strengths and weaknesses. The procedure takes less than an hour and is painless.

When your physician knows your glandular capacities, it is much easier to help you regain your health. As described earlier, the hormones released by these glands are powerful chemicals that are responsible for our most basic bodily functions. If they are excreted in excess or in paltry amounts, things just don't work well inside.

If glandular imbalances are part of your health picture, all the improvements in your lifestyle will help to reestablish balance. Your new way of eating, regular exercise, refusal to take stressful drugs, attitude adjustment, and anti-yeast medication can benefit your glands. Often, as Candida dies off, the glands immediately show signs of improvement.

Specific nutrients may be prescribed to assist your glands. The adrenal glands are known to thrive on pantothenic acid and vitamin C. The thyroid gland needs iodine, found abundantly in kelp. Each gland needs certain nutrients to be healthy. Your physician can plan this supplement program for you.

In some cases, minute doses of the hormones produced by these glands are prescribed. Thyroid hormones are often recommended.

Research by Dr. Page revealed that 88 percent of

the chronically ill women that came to his clinic had genetically underactive posterior pituitary glands. He found that these women healed much more rapidly when they took posterior pituitary hormones in very small doses. A physician who studied the Page work or attended workshops conducted at the Page Clinic would be capable of prescribing these hormones and the complimenting nutrients.

What about toxic metals? There are many techniques for determining an excess accumulation of lead, mercury or cadmium. There is debate about the accuracy of each of these tests, so your physician may choose to do several different types of tests to see if the results correlate. Hair analysis, urine tests, blood analysis, tissue biopsies, signs and symptoms, your exposure to sources of these metals; any or all of these tests may be recommended.

As we have said earlier, silver dental fillings can be a built-in source of mercury. A mercury vapor test may be recommended by your doctor. Dentists who specialize in the replacement of silver fillings often have the equipment necessary for this testing. Your physician may refer you to such a dentist.

The mercury vapor test requires that you chew sugar free gum for five to ten minutes. This abrasive activity on the surface of your dental fillings can stimulate the release of mercury in the form of gas or vapor. A sensitive instrument is then held over your teeth to measure the amount of mercury vapor in your mouth.

If you have symptoms of mercury accumulation and high levels of mercury vapor being released from your fillings, your physician and dentist may recommend removal of the mercury and replacement with another material. A nutrient program, along with the diet and other health recommendations in this book, will enhance your body's ability to unload mercury and any other toxic metals.

If your tests show lead accumulation, you will want to investigate chelation therapy. This is the treatment of choice for lead toxicity and will also aid in the removal of any other heavy, toxic metals.

How do you know if circulation problems are a part of your Candida condition? Again, a physician is needed to make this determination.

A thorough physical examination is the first step in evaluating circulation. Signs, symptoms and your health history will yield some clues. Your doctor will also check the strength of your pulse at various points on your body.

By using ocular instruments to look into the eye ground, the condition of your retinal blood vessels is visible to the doctor. Anatomically, these are direct extensions of your brain. If these vessels in the retina of the eye are in great shape, it suggests the same about the blood vessels in your brain. If they are occluded, the assumption is that your cerebral blood vessels are in a similar condition.

To check the circulation below the brain, there are many techniques and instruments. One instrument is an oscillometer. This procedure requires less than thirty minutes of your time. It is neither painful nor toxic. The physician uses the oscillometric index from this examination to assess the quality of your blood flow.

Ultrasound is being used extensively for the diagnosis of cardiovascular problems. This testing involves no radiation, no insertion of needles and no chemicals. Unlike many of the tests performed in hospitals, there are no hazards to this technique. Many physicians now have this equipment in their offices, so it is unnecessary to go to a hospital for the evaluation.

The Doppler ultrasound device operates some- what like a dolphin. That's right, the sea mammal. Both rely on interpreting an echo to "see." Sonar signals at a range too high to be picked up by the human ear are used. These signals are transmitted, bounced off a target, then are received and trans- lated into a picture. This technique is used to study the condition of the arteries in the neck and within the skull. Echocardiography shows the condition of the heart.

To evaluate the circulation in the hands, feet, legs, or other body parts below the neck, a plethy- smograph may be used. This blood-pressure type of testing equipment measures the muscle tone and amount of blood volume of your arteries. It also tells your physician how fast your blood is moving. Like the other tests described here, this is abso- lutely nonhazardous and painless.

If you have circulation problems, reversing them is essential to your healing. Remember the rule of the artery. Only tissues with good blood supply can be truly healthy. Controlling Candida, like any other disease, is easier when your circulation contributes to the cure.

There is a broad spectrum of circulation-improving techniques. A good diet is important. The one in this book is ideal. Exercise works. Food supple- ments are beneficial. Meditation and visualization techniques make sense. For instance, in a relaxed state, see your arteries opening and clearing them- selves of plaque. Visualize increased blood flow to the diseased areas of your body.

An intravenous series of treatments, called chela- tion therapy, is often helpful in reversing circula- tory disease. There are several books on this subject. Check your local library or book store for *Bypassing Bypass* by Elmer M. Cranton, M.D.

EXERCISE: MOVEMENT TOWARD HEALTH

Health professionals disagree on the importance of diet, food supplements and the mercury in dental fillings. On the subject of exercise, there is little debate. Exercise is important to health.

Benefits of exercise are more than firm muscles, perfect weight and increased oxygen supply to your tissues. Psychologists are saying that exercise is sometimes as effective as therapy at relieving depression. Studies show that people who exercise regularly experience less anxiety in the drama of daily living.

Exercise was a concept our ancestors had no need for. Movement and muscle use was a way of life. Chopping wood, building the barn, chasing rabbits, picking berries, scrubbing clothes, churning butter, airing the mattress: aerobic activity was everywhere. In our recent past, manual typewriters, crank telephones and nonescalated stairs offered a little more activity than our current automated existence.

Today we live in a society that does not provide exercise as an integral part of living. Electric typewriters, telephone extensions, swivel chairs, golf carts, escalators—due to these conveniences, living requires very little movement. If we don't make exercise a conscious priority, it just doesn't happen.

For exercise to happen in your life, it must be carefully planned. If you have the fatigue that often accompanies diseases such as candidiasis, it's easy to excuse yourself from exercise. After all, you're too tired. Even if you know that exercise is important, it's usually your last priority. Soon it's the end of the day and you just didn't have the time to get around to it.

To keep your commitment to daily exercise, it helps to plan your day in advance. Each morning, make a written health plan for the day. Be very specific. Write down when you will eat. Use your list as a reminder to take your food supplements. Are meditation and prayer your natural tranquilizers? Write it down. Plan your exercise activity and the time at which you will do it.

As you go through the day, keep your list within reach. As you complete each item, write a C for completed after the item and cross it off the list. This is a way of patting yourself on the back for having kept your word. It won't be long before you'll be getting lots of pats on the back. Glowing health attracts admiration.

If you don't complete an activity, this is not the time to berate yourself. Guilt and blame do not inspire health. Before bed, look over your list. After the items you did not complete, write a T for transfer, draw a line through those items and be sure to add them to the next day's list.

Now you know how to fit exercise into your schedule. Your next step is to decide what kind of exercise is best for you. If you are extremely fatigued and unaccustomed to exercise, why not begin with walking? Walking from the recliner to the window might be a start. Going to the mailbox and back may be enough for your first few days. Rather than discredit yourself for not participating in an aerobics class or jogging two miles a day, credit yourself for having the intelligence to choose an activity that is appropriate for your current state of health. Even after your health is completely restored, you may continue to choose walking as your best exercise activity.

"Walking is the best exercise there is," according to Ronald M. Lawrence, M.D., medical advisor to the U.S. Olympic Committee and to the President's Council on Physical Fitness Sports. "It uses more of the body's muscles than any other type of exercise, improves cardiovascular efficiency and is virtually injury free." And, it can be done by almost anyone.

Walking has always been more popular than jogging. Now fitness experts say it is probably better for you. The injuries that runners experience—runner's knee, shin splints, groin pulls—are problems rarely faced by walkers.

By walking you can literally stroll into shape. Want to slim down? Like all exercise, walking decreases the appetite as well as it burns up calories. The backs and fronts of your legs can become sleeker, your calves and buttocks can be firmer, your hips slimmer. Since walking also works on the upper body, other benefits can be a firm abdomen and arms, and shapely shoulders and back.

It is common knowledge that walking helps the heart. Continuous and rhythmic, it forces the heart to pump more oxygenated blood through your body. As walking works the muscles below your waist, they relax and contract. This causes these muscles to act like a second heart. They force the blood back up from the lower body where it tends to pool when you are sitting or standing.

Did you know that walking is also good for your head? It relieves tension. The increased oxygen to the brain is lifting to the spirit. Walking enhances the production of neurotransmitters, the brain chemicals that have a mood elevating effect. Equally important to your brain is the centering effect of walking. When you allow your arms to swing free—unencumbered with purses or parcels—walking is a cross-crawl body movement. As your left leg moves out, your right arm moves out. Coordination of these opposite sides of the body results in coordination of the opposite hemispheres of the brain which in turn assists in glandular balance.

Walking does not require expensive equipment.

What do you need to get started? Comfortable clothes and good running or athletic shoes.

If walking does not appeal to you, there are many other activities from which to choose. Running or jogging is a quick calorie burning activity and a great leg, buttock and thigh firmer.

Biking provides fresh air, the thrill of speed and stronger legs, heart and lungs.

Swimming is the most symmetrical body toner, utilizing more muscles simultaneously than any other exercise. Since the body moves almost effortlessly in water, this workout is also relaxing. In fact, swimming is considered injury-proof. It is often prescribed to relieve aches and pains and to repair bad backs.

Aerobic or other exercise classes are offered at YMCAs, health clubs and community centers. This exercise activity offers the most for the body in the shortest time. The classes deal with abdominal strength, firm thighs, trim waists and flat stomachs. As with all exercise, release from nervous tension is a big payoff.

Yoga is often associated with gentle souls who are interested in spiritual exploration and are patient and non-competitive. Yoga has a tranquilizing effect on the mind. Done properly, it is non-traumatic to novices who are out of shape. It has been known to lower blood pressure, improve digestion and relieve headaches. Excellent teachers can be found in health clubs, colleges and private classes.

Dance is a form of exercise in which one can pour out emotions in movement. Dance also produces poise, good posture, elastic muscles, great legs, flat stomachs and cardiovascular fitness.

Weight training is the quickest way to remodel your arms, legs and torso. You will see improvements in two weeks! Weight training not only allows you to design and mold your shape, it also develops concentration and discipline. If movements are done in sufficient repetition, this activity can also be aerobic.

Tennis, racquetball and team sports provide camaraderie as well as exercise. These competitive sports are great for buttocks, legs, arms, wrists and hand-eye coordination.

Once you've selected the perfect exercise for you, continue to exercise that old stand-by, common sense. If you have serious health problems and develop symptoms or complaints at low activity levels, see a physician before beginning any exercise program. If your program requires a teacher, find a good one. Whatever you choose to do, begin slowly. Above all, forget the adage, "No Pain, No Gain!" Listen to your body talk. Pain can usually be translated as "Stop!"

What can be translated as "Keep it up!"? Firmer muscles, increased stamina and awareness of energy and fitness, the satisfaction of having comfortably completed an activity that may have seemed impossible when you first considered it. Soon you may find that you are looking forward to the activity that you once dreaded. Acknowledge that you have broken through your resistance. Enjoy the opportunity to see your determination, commitment to health and your strength in action.

HOUSEHOLD MOLDS:
PUTTING YOUR HOUSE IN SHAPE

Candida overgrowth often sets up a sensitivity to common molds that live in our homes and gardens. They are incapable of causing diseases, but once the immune system is weakened, allergic reaction to these molds is common.

Dampness and darkness inspire molds to grow profusely. A basement is the perfect spot. The spores produced there can steadily float upstairs and drift around the house. If you are a pack rat, the basement is probably where you're hoarding all those old newspapers, magazines, books and clothes. These provide a perfect growth medium for mold.

A dehumidifier will help retard basement mold growth. The control setting on the humidifier can be placed at a lower level than in areas of your home where you spend lots of time. An automatic, large-capacity dehumidifier is preferable. This model will shut off when the humidity drops to the designated level.

The dehumidifier itself can become the perfect home for molds, so clean it at least once a week. If you use chemicals to clean this equipment, they will be released into the air and then inhaled by your family. Scrub the dehumidifier without using chemicals. A stiff vegetable brush and water will do the job.

Is your basement noticeably more damp after a rain? If so, maybe the roof downspout is too close to the house. Water is being deposited very close to the foundation. A simple solution here is to extend the leader to carry the water further away from the house. This extension can deposit the water so that it runs away from the basement.

Your bathroom is another popular residential area for molds. The caulking between shower tiles and between the tub and the wall is an ideal medium. The shower curtain is another good place. The floor behind the toilet is a secluded area where molds often go unnoticed. Regular cleaning of bathrooms is an obvious solution. Another solution to the overall problem is to improve air circulation. A built-in shower exhaust will handle this issue.

The kitchen is also a hospitable area for molds. A mold colony usually settles under the sink at the damp, dark junction of sink and wall. Borax, the natural bleach that is used in washing clothes, can be sprinkled in this area to prevent mold growth.

The surplus water tray under self-defrosting refrigerators is a mold center *par excellence*. Did you know that you had such a tray? If you have never seen this refrigerator attachment and you are getting ready to go into the kitchen and bravely pull it out from under the fridge, get ready for a mold-a-mania: a fuzzy, furry, splotchy scene may await you. This tray should be emptied and cleaned regularly with borax.

The soil in houseplants is often a source of mold spores. The soil surfaces can be covered with a layer of little stones and this will limit mold dispersal.

Closets harbor mold. During the warm, humid summer months, you may want to leave the light on in your closet. At night, the door can be left ajar to provide fresh air. Clothes and shoes that are saturated with perspiration invite mold growth.

Even mattresses and pillows can house mold. Avoid going to bed with wet hair and letting the water soak into your mattress or pillow. Wash the mattress pad regularly.

Molds in your yard or garden produce spores which waft into your home. Mulch such as dried leaves, lawn clippings and hay yield generous mold communities. If your garden is downwind of your house, you are in luck.

When you are healthy is the time you are really "in luck." Then, you will not be sensitive to these useful molds of nature, which are not there to cause reactions, but to recycle and decompose organic matter.

DRESS FOR HEALTH

The ideal growth climate for yeasts is a warm, moist place. Female genitalia have all the qualifications. Add pantyhose, tight jeans, polyester slacks, nylon panties, sweat suits and nylon exercise leotards and you have just created the perfect growth medium for Candida albicans. These pieces of clothing restrict air circulation to the vagina, making it even warmer and locking in moisture.

If you do not have vaginitis or Candida overgrowth in the vaginal area, dressing this way may not be a problem. If you do have vaginitis, look at alternative ways of dressing that will support your healing.

Buy pantyhose with a cotton crotch or switch to garter belts and stockings. Buy cotton panties instead of nylon ones. You like lacy feminine undies? They're making those styles in cotton.

Tight jeans and polyester slacks will best be avoided in hot weather. They provide no air space and little circulation. Polyester fabric does not "breathe." Heat and moisture are locked in.

Sweat suits and nylon exercise leotards should be removed immediately after your exercise session. Cotton exercise leotards are a healthier alternative to nylon ones, but should still be removed if they are wet with perspiration after a workout.

Sitting around in a wet bathing suit also encourages continued yeast problems. If you want to stay around the pool after a swim, slip into cotton panties and loose fitting cotton shorts.

Men occasionally have fungus growth on their genitalia. If so, you need to wear loose fitting boxer shorts, not the tight jockey style. Jockey shorts raise the temperature in the genital area and obviously restrict the flow of air.

Natural fabrics, such as cotton or linen, would be the ideal material for your pants. Loose fitting trousers have been in style for several years and are a much healthier choice than tight-fitting jeans or snug polyester slacks.

ATTITUDINAL HEALING

> The care of tuberculosis depends more on what the patient has in his head than what he has in his chest.
>
> SIR WILLIAM OSLER

This section is last in the chapter on restoring your health because it is the least important, right? Wrong! This sequence illustrates, "Save the best for last."

Why is this section the best? Because it is the area of the most exciting discoveries. It is also the most powerful. Without healing your attitude, nothing else presented in this book will work. Diet might work for a while, but unless your attitude is working with it, you won't stay on the diet. Anti-yeast drugs might keep things under control temporarily, but unless you let your attitude help with the job, even drugs become ineffective.

The first step may be simply to listen to yourself. Do you tell others that you are a "victim" of candidiasis? Are you being "attacked" by yeasts and molds? Are you "flattened" by petrochemical fumes? Is "I'm *trying* to get better," said with a distinct whine, your motto? The word *try* implies effort, struggle and eventual failure. Is that what you really want for yourself?

Victim, attacked, flattened, try—all of these words insinuate helplessness, loss of power. That's the way you feel? Okay, so play a little game. This game is called Make It Up. When you first begin to play this game you will probably laugh at yourself. The things you say will sound so foolish that you'll find them amusing.

Start with, "I am not a victim. I am a powerful person!" When you say this, you could be lying flat on your back, too weak to move beyond the nightstand. But no matter. Continue.

It will take a while for you to believe that you are powerful. Everytime the little voice says, "I am a victim," you might counter aloud with, "Cancel that thought. I am actually powerful." If biblical evidence carries any weight, refer to II Timothy 1:7. "For God has not given us a spirit of fear, but of power and of love and of a sound mind."

To weaken your spirit of fear, do not refer to yourself as having been attacked. Why not say, "I reacted to the mold." Are you actually "flattened" by petrochemical fumes? Are you really prone beside the highway, horizontal on the pavement? If so, here's an excellent chance to see just how advanced you have already become in the game of Make It Up. You might say, "These fumes have given me an opportunity to rest for a moment."

This game is also a vitamin deficiency test. If you aren't laughing by now, you need more B vitamins.

This business of words may sound silly, but making up new and more effective ways of talking about yourself and talking to yourself can be the beginning of your healing process.

Speaking of process, that's the next issue to be examined. You probably became diseased, weak and debilitated over a period of time, not overnight. That's most likely how your healing will occur too—gradually, not in an instant. It will be a healing process. If you set up rigid expectations, such as "by next Friday, all my symptoms will be gone, I'll be running four miles a day, back to work, and fifteen pounds lighter," you may be setting yourself up for disappointment.

Make your expectations work for you. Why not say, "I expect a miracle!" and then see every little step in your process to radiant health as a miracle. You could walk around the block! That's a miracle if you had not made it past the mailbox in three months. To chronicle your progress, keep a healing journal. Write down every improvement, no matter how small. If you don't record these changes, you will probably forget how far you've come. The mind can forget past pain quickly. When you get discouraged, read your journal. This is evidence that you are on the mend.

When you feel discouraged, don't attempt to hide those feelings. Let them out. Crying is one of the best ways to let go of sadness, disappointment, anger and fear. The calmness and peace after a good cry is reminiscent of the stillness and serenity that follows a violent storm. Let your storms rage and then subside.

It helps to have some healthy friends. These people can remind you of the possibilities available to you. If most of your friends are also ill, enroll them in the game of Make It Up. If, instead, you get together to compare severity of symptoms and commiserate on the desperation of life, you can be dragged back down into chronic illness as if by quicksand.

There is one special type of friend that can help pull you up from the quicksand. This friend has been there. This is the person who has been very ill and has turned it around. This person is not bitter, but grateful for the opportunity to learn how to live more effectively. This person may not yet be in perfect health but is clearly headed in that direction. This person who patiently participates in the healing process, can be your mentor, your encouragement, your example. Let that person give you support and love.

Letting love in may be one of the most significant break-throughs in your healing process. Many of us decided very early in life that we were unlovable. We may have interpreted our parents' unhappiness as an indication that we weren't good enough. Those early declarations, "I'm not good enough" or "I don't deserve love" may be phrases that we continue to repeat unconsciously. It's difficult to accept love when, deep inside, you're insisting that you don't deserve it.

If you're experiencing health problems, that's even more evidence that you aren't good enough. How could anyone so helpless, weak, skinny, fat or unproductive deserve love?

Time for the Make It Up game. Say to yourself, out loud, "I am good enough." Then add, "I deserve love." Write these phrases repeatedly and allow the wisecracks to come out too. "You? I thought justice was at work in the universe." Keep writing until all your arguments against self-love are dispelled. This may take months. Let that be okay.

To reinforce these new ideas about yourself, write affirmations on colorful paper and put them in your bathroom, on your refrigerator door, on the wall in front of your bed. Along with "I deserve love." you might add, "Expect a miracle." and "I enjoy this healing process."

If you believe in God, there are powerful verses from the Bible and other spiritual writings that can go up on your wall. "The Lord is my shepherd, I shall not want." "I am with you always." "The Lord is wondrous kind."

Keep a treasure map in your mind's eye, available at any time, in any place you find yourself. Are you on the subway, having a reaction to the perfume sitting beside you? Quick! See yourself inhaling the breeze that gently blows across the lagoon on this South Sea island where you are lying on the beach. You are bathed in a pink glow, warmed by the sun that evaporates all your pain, all your troubles. This is another phase of Make It Up. The first phase is saying what you want. Now you are seeing what you want.

It takes courage to play these games. It goes against logic. It is beyond understanding. Does anyone understand how visualization works? There has not been a double-blind study to validate the power of belief or the effectiveness of treasure maps.

Acknowledge your courage and determination to do what it takes to regain your health. Your acknowledgement carries more weight than that of others. Acknowledge yourself for taking a walk, staying on your diet for three days, remembering to take your supplements. Acknowledge your sense of humor, your ability to care about others when you are in need of care yourself. Put yourself up, not down.

Forgiveness plays a central role in putting yourself up. Forgiveness is a good word to add to your treasure map. Write "I forgive myself completely." repeatedly in your healing journal and see what comes up. Guilt and self-directed anger are blocks to healing.

While you're handling forgiveness, remember to include your mother, father and everyone else in your life. Dead or alive, everyone counts. Anger and resentment against others boomerang, and eat away at your self-love, chip away at your self-esteem.

If you believe in God, asking Him for forgiveness

and then receiving it can be the ultimate boost to your self-esteem. If God says you're okay, is there anyone else with whom that issue has to be discussed?

Suppose God has a purpose for your life. Ready for the ultimate fantasy? Maybe your illness and recovery is part of God's plan for your life. Could it be that some good is coming from all this misery? Maybe you are learning valuable lessons. Maybe you will share these lessons with others. Is it possible that you had to get low to get high? Maybe you are learning to trust the ultimate goodness and purpose of the universe.

Just a few years ago these ideas were not "in" at all. Self-reliance was the theme song. There was even a rumor that God had died. It was in vogue to be cynical, to demand proof for everything.

Now even scientists are admitting that there are lots of important beliefs about things that we can't literally see. Gravity is a good example. We see its effects, but we never see it. Electrons appear to be around, but one has never actually appeared—that is, no human has ever seen one. Yet most people believe in electrons.

Faith is belief in something unseen. Prominent health professionals are citing the Faith Factor as very important to the healing process. If it is not faith in God it is a faith in the healing process.

Herbert Benson, M.D., who has credentials such as Associate Professor of Medicine, Harvard Medical School, wrote a popular and controversial book several years ago. *The Relaxation Response* affirmed the healing potential in the practice of meditation at a time when meditation was being relegated to the ravings of hippie communes.

Recently, Dr. Benson took another brave stand. In his latest book, *Beyond the Relaxation Response*, he extolls the power of prayer in combination with meditation techniques. This book offers prayers for all major faiths such as Jewish, Christian, Hindu, Buddhist, Moslem. It offers prayers for people of no traditional religious belief. The Faith Factor can be reinforced by repetition of a neutral, non-religious word.

Before you disregard the idea of prayer as an insult to your intelligence, read Dr. Benson's book. Use the techniques for at least a week. If you are immobilized by candidiasis, you may not have a choice. At this point, inner serenity and balance may be your best lifeline.

Human touch is also a powerful lifeline. As an expression of love, touching can transmit messages at moments when words are not enough.

Leo Buscaglia has become the guru of touch, generously giving and receiving hugs as part of his presentation of love as healer. In a recent best seller, *Loving Each Other*, Buscaglia offers data for the proof that love affects health. He reminds us that touch deprivation often leads to loss of appetite, despondency and apathy. He cites a study linking an increase in blood hemoglobin levels with increased amounts of touching. Since hemoglobin is that segment of the blood that transports oxygen, increased levels strengthen all parts of the body, speed recovery from disease and bolster immunity.

We aren't the only mammals that seem to thrive on touching. In 1983, Ohio State University disclosed the results of controlled studies with rabbits. Those who were cuddled and held during feeding developed only half the arteriosclerosis as those who were not cuddled, even though both groups of rabbits had identical diets.

Does hugging relieve pain? Dr. David Bressler, former director of the Pain Control Unit at UCLA

Medical Center thinks so. He often writes an official prescription that says, "four hugs a day."

If you are feeling deprived, a victim of no hugging, guess who can change that immediately? You. Hugging takes two. It rarely is a result of simultaneous movements. One person usually initiates and the other responds. If you aren't getting hugged, that means you aren't hugging. Make the first move. The game of Make It Up can be revived. There are people coming across your path today who need to be hugged by you.

This emphasis on touching and hugging shows plainly that love is something that is transmitted from one person to another. However, the most profound love comes from within oneself with self-acceptance, self-esteem.

It has been said that the most healing sentence is, "I love you." Paradoxically, when you say that to others, you hear it for yourself. When you start giving love to others, you start getting it for yourself. When you sincerely acknowledge, love and forgive others, you find it easier to do those things for yourself. Soon, it flows effortlessly. In giving, you receive. In helping, you are helped. In forgiving, you are forgiven. In loving, you are loved. In helping others to heal, you are healed.

Serious stuff? It can be. That's where humor comes in. Enlightenment is a valuable part of your healing process. Remember that one definition of enlightenment is lightening up.

Laughter is still one of the best medicines. As an anti-yeast medication, it is unexcelled. If you have common symptoms of candidiasis—intestinal gas, bloating, memory loss—you are a rich source of humorous episodes. Giggle generously. Laugh at yourself before someone else beats you to it. This is phase three of Make It Up. Transform potential tragedy into comedy.

Counting your blessings is phase four of Make It Up. At first, you may recite things like "Clean sheets to lie on all day long." Keep going. Name every friend you ever had. Is there food in your refrigerator? You're ahead of lots of other people on the planet. Do you have enough money to pay your bills? Ahead again.

Gratitude is a very centering emotion. It brings with it a sense of joy and contentment. If you keep it up, you can eventually reach a point of happiness. In the face of gratitude, heavy, troublesome feelings flee. When you're focused on your blessings, worries can't even get a foot in the door.

If you are walking for exercise, this is a great time to name your blessings aloud, to repeat your self-acknowledgements, or to remind yourself whose child you are. As you walk, you can repeat brief phrases in cadence with your step. "I am healing." works well. "I forgive myself completely." is a good one. "I forgive my father completely" or "I forgive my mother completely." The list can go on and on.

Reading books which reinforce your attitudinal healing is extremely helpful. Just a few pages every day can make a big difference for you. Below is a list of well-worn books from my personal shelf:

> The Bible (the Book of Psalms is highly recommended).
>
> Benson, Herbert, *Beyond the Relaxation Response.*
>
> Buscaglia, Leo, *Living, Loving and Learning, Loving Each Other.*
>
> Cousins, Norman, *Anatomy of an Illness.*
>
> Dyer, Wayne, *Gifts from Eykis, Pulling Your Own Strings, The Sky's the Limit, Your Erroneous Zones.*

Gawain, Shakti, *Creative Visualization*.
Moscato, Tony, *You Bet You Can* (P.O. Box
        3302, Glendale, CA 91201).
Jampolsky, Gerald, *Love Is Letting Go of Fear*.
Ray, Sondra, *I Deserve Love*, *The Only Diet
        There Is*, *Loving Relationships*.
Schuller, Robert, *Self Esteem*, *Tough Times
        Never Last but Tough People Do*.

Weekend seminars and workshops that deal with
releasing guilt, letting in love, developing trust
and forgiveness and other important issues can be
miraculous in your healing process. These meetings
often include 100 to 200 people. That may sound
frightening and yet the opposite is true. These
groups can be the safest experience you have ever
had. The people in these groups are just like you
in that they are looking for solutions. They want
to grow. They are seeking more abundant health.
They want to feel comfortable and secure with
other human beings. They want to be loved and to
love.

Four of these seminars are listed here. These groups
offer weekend experiences in various cities all around
the country. To find out when and where one will
be offered in your area, call or write the centers
listed here below:

    Insight
    2101 Wilshire Boulevard
    Santa Monica, CA 90403
    (213) 829-9816

    Lifespring
    4340 Redwood Highway, Suite 50
    San Rafael, CA 94903
    (415) 479-7873

Loving Relationships Training
145 West 87 Street
New York, NY 10024
(212) 799-7323

Werner Erhard and Associates
765 California Street
San Francisco, CA 94108
(415) 391-9911

If you are too weak to attend a seminar, or you are reacting to newsprint and are unable to read, here's another alternative. Listen. There are many audio tapes currently available that can reinforce your healing attitude. If you spend much time in traffic, listen to these tapes along the way. If you spend lots of time in bed or in your recliner, invest in a tape player and some worthwhile messages.

Several excellent tape sets are listed below. These can be ordered from the Nightingale-Conant Corporation, 7300 North Lehigh Avenue, Chicago, Illinois 60648. Phone 1-800-323-5552 or (312) 647-0300.

Buscaglia, Leo, *Love*
Cousins, Norman, *Mind Over Illness*
Dyer, Wayne, *How to be a No-Limit Person*
Secrets of the Universe

VII CASE HISTORIES

FRAN

ACNE, BLOATING, FATIGUE, repeated urinary tract infections—none of these had motivated Fran, a thirty-one-year-old novelist, to call for an appointment at the Life Care Medical Center, Pompano Beach, Florida. She had learned to live with these signals. Her most recent signal, however, was more difficult to accept. Her hair was falling out in handfuls.

As with each new patient in which we suspect Candida overgrowth, an hour was devoted to reviewing her health history from infancy to the present. Correlating symptoms with dietary abuse, antibiotic therapy and use of the birth control pill, it was apparent that Candida was very likely a part of Fran's health crisis.

Since childhood, her diet had been heavily laced with chocolate, sweets and pizza. Recurrent ear and upper respiratory infections in childhood had prompted repeated rounds of penicillin. Acne, which began in adolescence and continued to the present, had evoked prescriptions for tetracycline. Menstrual cramps, yeast vaginitis, cystitis and more acne followed. Fran was now fatigued, both mentally and physically. Her creative thinking was almost at a standstill. She had not been able to begin work on the rewrite requested months earlier by her publisher.

After three weeks on a program of the diet outlined in this book and oral nystatin powder, Fran returned to report weight loss, a flat stomach, skin almost clear of acne, no more hair loss and a dramatic increase in energy. She was sleeping three hours less daily and awakening feeling rested. Her previous depression had been replaced by smiles, as she reported that she had resumed work on her rewrite and expected to send her novel to the publisher within the next month.

ERIC

Eric, a thirty-six-year-old interior designer, looked like an ad for the health spa he frequented. With regular workouts, he had produced enviable muscles. He was the proverbial picture of health. Looks were deceiving! Eric was plagued with headaches and fatigue. He had lost his taste for animal protein and preferred fruits, grains, dairy products and honey. He was fighting weight gain in spite of regular exercise and felt full and logy after meals. Sinusitis was frequent, bowel movements infrequent.

Candidiasis is more difficult to spot in men than in women. Since we were not sure of Eric's situation, we did not recommend use of nystatin. Several months of diet changes and supplementation did not significantly alter his symptoms, however, so a therapeutic trial was prescribed.

Weeks later, Eric returned for a follow-up visit. He began the interview by stating that he had never felt better in his life. He was having excellent bowel function, no more struggle with weight gain, a head free of aches and incredible energy. Most incredible to him was that his lifelong craving for sweets was gone. He now preferred animal protein and vegetables.

CAROLYN

When Carolyn returned to the U.S. after five years in Tanzania, Africa, she brought home more than the usual souvenirs. Chronic upper respiratory infections, extreme muscle weakness, rapid pulse, excess perspiration, difficulty breathing, constipation, eyes bulging slightly—Carolyn was a textbook case of hyperthyroidism. American doctors promptly suggested oblation with radioactive iodine. In other words, kill the overactive thyroid gland.

Carolyn preferred a less radical approach to her problems. She began doing some research and reading about alternatives. An article in *Let's Live* magazine featured the Page method of evaluating and supporting the glandular system. Carolyn's chiropractor, who had attended Page seminars for health professionals, recommended that she come to our clinic for evaluation and treatment.

The Page system allowed Carolyn to tone down her overactive thyroid gland naturally. First focus was on her diet. Foods to which she was sensitive were eliminated and she began eating the diet featured in this book. A Heidelberg Digestive Analysis revealed a deficiency of hydrochloric acid in the stomach and insufficient alkalinity in the small intestine. Digestive aids were prescribed until her system normalized.

Conversations with a psychologist revealed that Carolyn was anxious, agitated and depressed. Recognizing the need for counseling, Carolyn continued these meetings, and made rapid progress in dealing with issues she had never examined effectively.

Endocrine therapy was of major importance in this case. Insulin injections toned down the activity of thyroid hormones at their binding sites. A combination of testosterone and estrogen, in micro-doses, assisted her exhausted adrenal glands and allowed her thyroid gland to slow down. With the addition of pituitary hormones, her blood glucose levels became normal.

Daily walks on the beach, often with staff members, was the perfect exercise for Carolyn. Sea breezes, blue skies and postcard sunsets further encouraged this thirty-nine-year-old woman to relax into healing.

Frequent blood and urine testing monitored Carolyn's progress. Hormone doses were fine-tuned and vitamin and mineral supplements were adjusted to her unique needs.

Muscle weakness continued to be a problem and in spite of normal blood glucose levels, Carolyn continued to crave carbohydrates. It was difficult for her to avoid overeating rice and other grains. Investigating her health history in even greater detail, doctors suspected chronic yeast overgrowth as part of her problem. Years of sugar consumption and stress in other areas of her lifestyle had set the stage for Candida albicans to set up housekeeping in Carolyn's body. Nystatin was prescribed. Almost immediately, food cravings began to subside. Muscle strength returned.

Carolyn had a chronic ear infection with nagging pain that had persisted for months. She mixed a little nystatin with distilled water and began putting drops of this mixture into her ear. Within twenty-four hours the pain was noticeably less, and within a few days was completely gone.

One month had passed since Carolyn had arrived at our clinic. The doctors were now satisfied that her program had been adequately designed and she was advised to continue it at home, sending in regular blood tests to be reviewed.

These tests reveal that Carolyn is making remarkable process. The prior symptoms are gone. A bubbling personality and solid self-confidence have replaced depression and timidity. She reports that the quality of her relationships with family and friends surpasses anything she thought possible. Fearing, just a few months ago, that she could never work again, she is now preparing résumés for a new career. Although she was previously plagued by fatigue, she now participates in a daily exercise class.

MARGARET

One weekend Margaret had driven the forty miles from Miami to Pompano Beach and had checked into an oceanfront motel. She had to get away from the pressures of work and home. Her exhaustion was real. Once checked in, she spent the entire weekend in bed—never walking the twenty yards to the private beach and gentle surf.

On the nightstand was a magazine with an article featuring Orian Truss, M.D., the allergist who first noticed the significance of Candida albicans overgrowth. As she read the article on Candida she felt as if her life history was being told. Returning home, she called Dr. Truss. He referred her to the Life Care Medical Center in Pompano.

Luckily, the appointment following Margaret's had been cancelled. More time than usual was needed to record her complex health history. At the age of thirty, Margaret had "felt like an old woman." Now, at fifty-one, she felt that she could barely go on. Headaches, sinus congestion, chronic sore throat, repeated bouts with pleurisy and asthma, bloating, diarrhea, endometriosis, kidney and bladder infections, numbness and tingling in arms and legs, rash and itching, sensitivity to sunlight. It was no surprise that she also named depression as one of her problems. Arthritic-like pains affected most of her joints and the pain in her chest made breathing a chore.

"Do you often wish you were dead and away from it all?" was one of the questions asked of Margaret on the Cornell Medical Index. She had circled yes.

A review of her diet showed that Margaret craved sweets, especially chocolate, and regularly ate milk, cheese, coffee, bread and wine. She smoked one pack of cigarettes daily.

Repeated respiratory infections had resulted in repeated rounds of antibiotic therapy. Tetracycline had been a staple in Margaret's diet. Birth control pills also had a home in her medicine chest. Nystatin powder and proper diet was prescribed with the agreement that she would return in five days for reevaluation.

Within just five days, Margaret noticed less bloating, no tightness in her throat, much less pain in her joints and disappearance of the pain in her chest. Fatigue was greatly diminished. For the first time in months, she had summoned the energy to go grocery shopping alone.

Nine days later, more improvements were noted. When a virus made the rounds at her office, she was much less affected than the other employees. Margaret celebrated this as a sign that her immune system was gaining strength.

Each visit revealed more significant progress in her healing. Congestion in her head went away;

stomach problems subsided and Maalox medication was discontinued. Soon, her sense of humor made a comeback. On her first few visits, she had cried. Now, the staff looked forward to her bantering wit and quick laughter.

The doctor had prescribed a full complement of vitamins and minerals as part of Margaret's program. She continued these, the diet, the nystatin powder, and added light exercise to her schedule.

Ten weeks after her first visit to our clinic, Margaret completed the Cornell Medical Index again so that we could measure her progress. This questionnaire asks 195 questions which denote signs and symptoms of disease. On the first visit, Margaret had answered yes to 107 questions. Now, positive responses had dropped to 32. In just ten weeks on an anti-Candida health program, 75 signs and symptoms of disease had vanished!

WAYNE

This thirty-three-year-old painting contractor thought that he was coming to the Life Care Medical Center for treatment of hypoglycemia. He was troubled with spells of complete exhaustion and sudden mood changes. He had a history of high blood pressure and heart palpitations. He complained of shaking and trembling. Occasionally, he would awaken during the night in a severe soaking sweat.

These symptoms he could tolerate. But dizziness and sensations of fainting were intolerable. Wayne was a roof cleaner and painter. His business involved walking on the roofs of houses. Not a place to feel dizzy or faint.

Physical examination revealed boils and pimples covering his back and shoulders, a problem that had been with him for decades. Chronic acne, beginning in his teenage years, had been treated with liberal amounts of antibiotics. Tetracycline had been the usual prescription, but during the past seventeen years, Wayne had regularly taken eight to ten types of antibiotics. Recently, prednisone had also been prescribed.

A lifestyle evaluation revealed that Wayne exercised regularly, aside from the physical activity at work. His diet included lots of cheese, and fruit was a favorite food.

Wayne's work was of special interest to the doctor. Florida tile roofs are exposed to lots of moisture and heat. Mildew, fungus and mold are the bane of the homeowner. Every couple of years, someone like Wayne is hired to spray clean the gray-black mold off and repaint the tile roof. Inhaling the mold spores released during high-pressure spray cleaning might not be a problem for everyone, but for someone with Wayne's history of antibiotic usage, mold allergy was likely to exist.

The doctor suggested that Wayne wear a protective mask at work. Dietary changes were recommended along with a therapeutic trial of nystatin.

Diagnosis of candidiasis is often made as a result of a therapeutic trial of this type. If the patient has symptoms of yeast overgrowth and a history of pro-yeast drug usage, an anti-yeast diet and anti-yeast medication can result in quick improvement. This improvement suggests that Candida overgrowth is a factor in this patient's health condition.

Wayne was a textbook case. Within weeks he noted significant improvement. The numbness in his arm subsided. His energy returned. He no longer had daily headaches. The boils and pimples on his back began to heal.

Several weeks later, Wayne called in a state of panic. His symptoms were all returning! Careful questioning cleared away any mystery. Feeling confident that he was on the mend, Wayne had deviated from the diet of fresh vegetables, whole grains and protein. He had resumed his former diet of cheese, fruit, nuts and yeast bread.

This was a valuable lesson. It is difficult for most Candida patients to realize that fruit, cheese and bread—all hyped as health foods—can be stressful during yeast overgrowth. It is especially difficult in the initial phases of treatment because cravings for these foods are often stronger than logic.

Our staff reassured Wayne that this dietary deviation was merely a detour in his healing process. He decided to water fast for two days and then resume the anti-yeast diet.

Sometimes, a brief fast is a good way to get off a phase of binge eating or dietary indiscretions. Many patients find that a one- or two-day water fast with nystatin leaves them with a feeling of balance and control that they previously lacked.

JEANETTE

At the age of forty-three, Jeanette found herself without a husband and with two children to support. Her teaching job did not provide adequate income so she began working at a department store on weekends. Soon she was promoted to weekend manager. Working seven days a week brought in more than money. It also yielded fatigue, resentment and anger. With no time for recreation, Jeanette's health began to deteriorate.

Deterioration was rapid and severe. Cancer was diagnosed in her lymphatic system and surgery was performed to remove the tumor and malignant tissues from her left leg.

Jeanette began to reevaluate the way she had chosen to live her life. Sensing that a lack of forgiveness was at the core of her problems, she began letting go of the anger and resentment she had harbored. She forgave her parents, her former husband and a recent lover. She also forgave herself.

For eight years following her surgery, Jeanette experienced no significant health problems—only recurring athlete's foot. Then, her left leg began swelling intermittently. It often happened after she drank wine. The bloated and swollen leg soon showed signs of infection. Her doctors ordered hospitalization and antibiotic therapy.

The swelling, bloating and infection cycle occurred every three months for three years. Every three months Jeanette took a series of antibiotics, usually Keflex or tetracycline.

What was going on? Three years prior to her first infection, Jeanette had become a traveling sales representative for a food supplement manufacturer. Visiting health food stores daily, she had learned much about better ways of eating. Sugar was no longer a regular in her diet. Fruit juices, fruit, cheese, whole grain breads, dried fruit and nut mixes and sprouts took care of many of her meals. On the road, she would frequently eat in restaurants, and at night occasionally enjoy a glass of wine to relax.

Jeanette had tried every vitamin supplement, amino acid, chelated mineral and enzyme on the shelves of the stores she visited. Bee pollen, oil of evening primrose, cod liver oil, exotic herbal combinations—everything but essence of unicorn whiskers—was in her cache.

In spite of all these supplements and what she thought was an excellent diet, recurring infections were the result. What could it be?

When she read an article on Candida albicans, Jeanette saw light at the end of her tunnel. It all began to fall into place. She had taken many drugs which stimulate yeast growth: antibiotics, steroids, the Pill. Foods containing yeast and mold were a problem for her, resulting in bloating, memory loss and sudden exhaustion. She had noticed these symptoms developing after drinking wine, eating cheese and enjoying smoked sausage. She could gain five pounds overnight after eating these yeasty foods.

The physician recommended necessary changes in diet and anti-yeast medication—nystatin powder. Improvement was swift. Nystatin and diet therapy were continued for several months.

In the past two years, since Jeanette eliminated dairy products, wine, yeast bread and fruit from her diet, infection in her leg has not occurred. During this time, she has taken no antibiotics, steroids or birth control pills.

Now Jeanette sees her bloating as an early signal to get her health procedures back into line. If she deviates from her diet, especially if she eats smoked food or fruit, the reaction is immediate. Bloating and mental fogginess is apparent. During these periods, she resumes nystatin therapy and adheres strictly to her diet.

Jeanette also sees this as a time to clear away toxic emotions. She forgives herself for having eaten foods she knew would be stressful.

Jeanette's current philosophy is one which would serve many of us. She states that forgiveness is the key to her new found health. Her commitment is to balance, not extremes. Into a busy day, she schedules prayer and meditation, swimming, sensible eating, moderate food supplementation, and interaction with supportive friends. It must be working. At fifty-three, Jeanette looks thirty-three!

DR. JONES

It was humiliating—an embarrassment to himself and his wife. Every night, at approximately 2:00 A.M., Dr. Jones dragged himself from bed, pulled on a pair of slacks over his pajamas, and sped to the all-night grocery store. Roaming the aisles like a madman, he threw eclairs, pickles, smoked fish, and ice cream into the cart. Unable to wait to feast at the kitchen table, he spread the items on the car seat, tore into a couple of wrappers, and began an engorgement that would end when the food did.

This had gone on for years and the couple was concerned. Dr. Jones was well educated, a prominent professional in Fort Lauderdale. His behavior made no sense.

For two years now, weekly psychotherapy had been the attempted solution. The psychiatrist suggested that guilt was driving Dr. Jones to behave in such a self-destructive way. Once the guilt was alleviated, he would sleep through the night. Guilt-laden events included early childhood behavior, teenage years and a divorce. Working through these complex circumstances could take many more years on the couch.

At a party attended by a staff member of the Life Care Medical Center, Dr. Jones' wife joked self-consciously about her husband's behavior. Beneath the nervous laughter, there was obvious worry.

Taking her aside, our staff member asked if she or Dr. Jones had ever heard of Candida albicans. Explaining that its overgrowth often created almost insatiable cravings for sweets and pickled foods, she suggested that Dr. Jones come in for an evaluation. Skeptically, the couple agreed to check out the possibility of candidiasis.

Samples of Dr. Jones' stool and scrapings from his throat were sent to the lab for yeast cultures to be grown. Unwilling to base a diagnosis on history, symptoms and a trial of diet and medication, Dr. Jones wanted traditional medical proof. Before he gave up sugar and pickles, he wanted to see scientific evidence that Candida had really overgrown.

These cultures do not always appear to be accurate. Patients who make great improvement on the anti-Candida program and thrive after anti-yeast medication often show no sign of Candida in a stool, throat or vaginal culture. We eagerly awaited the results of Dr. Jones's lab work.

"Heavy Candida albicans growth in stool culture. Heavy Candida albicans growth in throat culture," read the laboratory report. Mrs. Jones beamed and clapped her hands. Dr. Jones slumped with a sigh. Could it be that there was some physiological basis for his bizarre nightly behavior?

Immediately, Dr. Jones began the anti-yeast diet. Days later, he added nystatin powder to the protocol. Taking 1/16 teaspoon of the yellow powder four times daily seemed to work. Several days later, he began sleeping through the night. Food cravings subsided and two weeks went by with no nightly trips to the grocery store.

As an unexpected fringe benefit of this health program his chronic sinus congestion disappeared. As an expected benefit he was twelve pounds lighter in two weeks.

Rapid loss of excess weight is common during reversal of candidiasis. Loss of bloating is significant with facial bones reappearing and ankles taking shape. The food cravings of candidiasis are for the fattening foods. No one ever dreams of celery sticks; it's usually ice cream or peanut butter.

Dr. Jones saw rapid and distinct improvement in his health. But he missed his cheese and bagels and pickles. Nighttime television wasn't the same without cookies. He slowly sneaked these items back into his diet. He discontinued the nystatin and food supplements.

Within two weeks, the weight was back, the sinus congestion had returned, and Dr. Jones was again a regular nocturnal customer at the twenty-four-hour grocery. During the past two years, he has not returned to our clinic for further assistance.

LINDA

She had been a fussy and colicky baby, wanting to nurse incessantly. Later, she experienced frequent colds, was a poor sleeper and could never seem to be still. Not quite classified as hyperactive, Linda definitely qualified as difficult. She was often defiant to adults and authority figures, especially parents and teachers. Initially, Mrs. T. had fed her children the typical American diet of sugared cereal, toast and jelly, soft drinks and cookies. But as she learned more about nutrition, she switched to what seemed to be healthier choices: fresh fruit, commercial yogurt with preserved fruit added, cheese. Cookies and ice cream were relegated to rare occasions. She added vitamins to the family's diet.

In spite of these dietary changes, Linda continued to have problems. She missed school frequently. When she was in school, there were reports from the teacher of her obstinate attitude and unwillingness to cooperate.

One year ago, a physician performed laboratory work—blood and urine testing—and informed Mrs. T. that Linda appeared to have a chronic yeast infection. To combat Candida overgrowth, nystatin powder and a diet of vegetables, whole grains and protein was advised. The physician was very clear in what should not be eaten: sweets, including fruit and fruit juice; cheeses; milk and the fruity yogurt the family had come to love; yeast bread.

At first, Linda whined and moaned. Orange juice is a staple in the diet of most Floridians. She had come to expect it every morning. Water was not an exciting substitute. Taking a lunch to school was a chore. Her food looked nothing like the other kids' bags of sandwiches and cookies, with milk or punch. At seven, one wants to be like everyone else.

The payoff soon made the diet more attractive. Linda stopped developing her regular colds. Her grades improved tremendously. Teachers began to praise her behavior. She continued the nystatin powder for eight weeks and maintained the diet, with infrequent deviation.

Looking back over the year, her mother rates the biggest changes in Linda's personality. "Linda is such a different little girl when she adheres to the yeast-free diet. If I want to remember the way she use to be, I just let her have something sweet. Within twenty minutes, she is transformed into a little monster!"

When Linda avoids the yeast-stimulating foods, she appears to be contented and congenial. She does not demand to have her own way and is willing to compromise.

Linda's father does not support his wife in maintaining the diet. He likes sweets and sometimes takes Linda and her sister out for pancakes and syrup, ice cream and soda. After these events, Linda's behavior is predictable. She becomes surly, irritable. Three days later she usually develops cold-like symptoms with thick green mucous discharge from her nose.

In spite of these occasional slip-ups, Linda's yeast-controlling year has paid off. She still has some difficulty with hand-eye coordination and does not do well in penmanship. If grades in that subject had been a little higher, she would have made the honor roll during every grading period this school year. That was a scholastic breakthrough.

CHERYL

Her childhood diet was similar to most that we have heard—sweets and penicillin. Frequent ear infections and years of intestinal worms had kept the family doctor busy. Teenage years were uneventful in terms of health. The usual pimples.

After her first baby, when she was twenty, the real trouble started. Severe depression and fatigue did not go away after the post-partum period ended.

Cheryl could barely cope with rearing her little boy. The couple agreed they would not have another child soon. Cheryl chose to have an IUD inserted.

For the next five years, vaginal problems reigned. Infections seemed never ending. A heavy discharge, itching and burning took Cheryl back to her physician regularly. He assured her that this was normal with the IUD. The answer was antibiotics. Keflex was often prescribed, and often sometimes tetracycline.

Cheryl had read a few books on nutrition and had eliminated refined sugar from the diet of her family. Now they put honey on their cereal, ate dried fruit and nuts instead of candy, often had fruit flavored yogurt for snacks.

When little Billy was two, Cheryl quit her job, unable to cope with the responsibilities of career and family. She was moody, had frequent headaches, chronic back pain and persistent nausea. Finally, her doctor recommended hospitalization and two weeks of testing. At the end of the stay, the physician revealed that nothing seemed abnormal.

The tests indicated that Cheryl was a healthy young woman.

She continued to seek answers. Another doctor diagnosed hypoglycemia and she went on the low carbohydrate diet touted during those years. Initially, there was improvement. Cheryl returned to work. The improvement did not last. After fainting on the job, she decided to visit a different doctor.

This new physician suspected candidiasis. Cheryl's history of vaginal infections and heavy antibiotic consumption rang lots of bells. He prescribed nystatin in relatively substantial doses—one teaspoon four times daily.

Although this physician was aware of Candida and the value of anti-yeast medication, he was not accurately informed on the subject of diet. He advised Cheryl to eat lots of fruit, especially when her energy flagged.

Years ago, this situation was common. It was not usually understood that fruit sugar is still sugar, and it can nurture yeast colonies.

While Cheryl was taking generous amounts of nystatin and simultaneously eating large quantities of fruit, she became very sensitive to chemicals. Automobile exhaust now brought on nausea and dizziness. Perfumes and deodorants seemed to impair her breathing and bring on immediate exhaustion. Foods to which she had never before reacted now seemed to evoke headaches, moodiness, fatigue. Even butter seemed to be a problem. Was it a dye or preservative to which she was sensitive? Thinking that nystatin might be somehow contributing to the sensitivities, Cheryl discontinued use of the drug.

After years of seeing physicians from Florida to Pennsylvania, Cheryl was referred to a health professional who advised a simple program: the diet featured in this book and light exercise. Having once been a dentist, he was aware of the potential of mercury toxicity from dental fillings. He looked into Cheryl's mouth. It was heavily adorned with silver.

A dental discussion followed. The year Cheryl's serious problems began was the year in which she had gotten six new silver fillings. Was it a coincidence that her health problems began that same year? The counselor's advice seemed sensible. Replace the silver fillings with a non-metal material and see what happens. There was a chance it could make a difference.

Within weeks after half of the mercury was removed from Cheryl's mouth, reactions to chemicals began to subside. In amazement, she began to say at every turn, "Nothing happened!" She ate in a restaurant, nothing happened. She inhaled cigarette smoke, nothing happened. She ate a candy bar, full of dyes, preservatives and sugar—nothing happened.

For the past six years, Cheryl and her husband had wanted to have another baby. It seemed impossible. Specialists had all agreed. Forget it. Too much scar tissue, too many complications. The couple had undergone extensive testing. Cheryl had endured painful procedures in an attempt to open her tubes. It looked final. Billy was to be their only child.

Shortly after the removal of her last mercury filling, Cheryl's health soared. She had noticed significant improvement after a few weeks on the anti-Candida diet. This, however, was a giant leap. High, steady energy was the rule, not the exception. Food cravings ceased. Vaginal symptoms cleared.

Ready for the fairy tale ending? Within a month after the removal of her last amalgam filling, Cheryl and her husband conceived a child. Now in her sixth month of pregnancy, she reports glowing health.

Looking back on the past ten years of illness, she

labels it simply a nightmare. But there is not a trace of bitterness. She is full of gratitude for having awakened.

GAIL NIELSON

In 1978, many women could have easily envied this pretty blonde who seemed to have it all—an adoring husband, a challenging career, two handsome, intelligent sons, and a home nestled in the hills of Castro Valley, California. A short time later, that envy would turn to sympathy.

As Gail swept the wood ashes off her porch one morning, hives began to appear on her skin. Within a few minutes, she gasped for air. She couldn't breathe. She was rushed to the nearby hospital where her life was saved by a quick shot of adrenaline.

The physician was puzzled by the incident. There seemed to be no logical explanation for what had just happened. Blood tests were analyzed and reviewed. Everything looked normal. Assuming the event to be psychosomatic, Gail's doctor advised her to deal with her psychological problems. His suggestion was to go out on the back porch and scream.

How could she scream when she couldn't breathe? Gail's respiratory attacks became frequent. She was taught to give herself the adrenaline shots when she felt the first symptoms of respiratory shutdown.

Other problems appeared. Stiffness and pain in her legs made walking difficult. Her hands soon became similarly affected. Knitting was now impossible. Then her eyes began to go and reading was out. Since thinking was also becoming difficult, Gail assumed her brain was deteriorating.

The first step in her recovery was a trip to a local allergist. This physician advised that she retreat to a rustic cabin, with few products of contemporary civilization. Taking along organically grown foods, Gail used her time at the cabin to test her reaction to these items. She ate one food at each meal and kept a record of any symptoms that developed after eating.

Back at home, Gail's husband was busy stripping the floor of synthetic carpets, removing plastics, discarding chemical cleaners and scented personal belongings. Even a metal telephone, used in the 1930s, was brought in to replace the modern plastic one.

This may sound ridiculous, but it is not to the thousands of Americans who are in the midst of what is termed "environmental illness." These people experience reactions which run the gamut from a headache to near-respiratory failure after exposure to chemicals or products which most of us consider to be innocuous: a little cigarette smoke, wallpaper glue, automobile exhaust, detergent residue in clothing.

As Gail learned early during her recovery, Candida albicans is often a factor in weakening the immune system so that it cannot cope with elements of ordinary life. Physicians have observed that many of these environmentally fragile people are carrying around toxin-producing colonies of Candida albicans.

For the first year and a half of her recovery period, Gail ate carefully, took the anti-yeast drug nystatin and bolstered her body chemistry with handfuls of vitamin and mineral supplements. She minimized her exposure to modern chemicals, making her own soap and ordering special natural fiber clothing.

Soon her eyesight had improved and she could read again. But she was still sensitive to the ink used in books, newspapers and magazines. This was easily solved. Her reading material was placed inside a metal box with a glass top. Holes in each side of the box were fitted with cotton gloves and Gail could turn the pages without direct exposure to the ink.

Progress was slow but steady. Gail recalls a leap forward in her healing when she began drinking taheebo tea, the herb reputed to strengthen the immune system and thus lead to yeast die-off. She began by drinking a few sips daily, then was soon drinking three to four cups of the amber colored brew.

Gail's regimen has paid off. Today, she is completely recovered. Watching this vibrant, beautiful woman cheerfully manage career, family and household chores, one would never guess that a few years ago, she was a sickly recluse.

To inform others of the Candida connection to environmental and other illnesses, Gail Nielson has formed the Candida Research and Information Foundation. This non-profit group of volunteers is affiliated with the Environmental Health Association of California and is committed to providing information on Candida-related diseases. A regularly published newsletter shares the latest findings with members of the organization. Patients are put in contact with other patients so that support groups can assist in the healing process. Meetings in Castro Valley feature speakers on Candida-related subjects.

For more information on the Candida Research and Information Foundation, send a self-addressed stamped envelope to: CRIF, P. O. Box 2719, Castro Valley, CA 94546 or phone (415) 582-2179.

VIII RECIPES

Appetizers

GUACAMOLE DIP

1 large ripe avocado or 2
   small ones, peeled and
   seeds removed
1 clove garlic
1 small white or red
   onion, chopped

juice of ½ lemon
½ teaspoon sea salt or
   kelp powder
¼ teaspoon chili powder
3 cherry tomatoes

Put all ingredients in a blender or food processor
and blend until smooth. Serve with crispy, raw vegetables or with yeast-free whole grain crackers. Delicious stuffed into celery sticks or hollowed out fresh
tomatoes.

Makes about 1½ cups.

BLACK BEAN ONION DIP

1 cup black beans,
   cooked
2 tablespoons olive oil
dash black pepper

½ cup white onions, finely
   chopped
¼ cup fresh parsley,
   chopped

Put ¾ cup of beans into blender or food processor with oil and black pepper. Add a little water or liquid from cooked beans if mixture is too thick. Blend well, pour mixture into bowl and stir in remaining beans. Place in serving bowl and sprinkle chopped onions atop bean dip. Use fresh parsley as a garnish.

Makes 1¼ cups.

MAYONNAISE

1 egg	¼ to ½ teaspoon salt,
2 tablespoons lemon	optional
juice	1 cup oil, room temperature

Break egg into blender and blend at low speed. Add lemon juice and salt, if desired. As you continue blending, slowly dribble in oil. Continue blending, adding oil slowly, until mayonnaise is thick and smooth. For extra pizzazz, add a clove of fresh garlic or a dash of curry powder.

Mayonnaise will remain fresh in the refrigerator for 2 to 3 days. This can serve as a salad dressing, vegetable dip or a fish sauce.

Makes 1 cup.

FROSTED TOMATOES

4 large ripe tomatoes	2 tablespoons fresh basil
1 small white onion, finely	leaves, finely chopped
chopped	salt and pepper, to taste

Peel tomatoes and grind or chop fine. Add onion, basil, salt and pepper to taste. Pour into shallow dish, cover and place in freezer for 1 to 2 hours. Leave in freezer until crystals of ice begin to form. Mixture should be mushy.

Serve in chilled glass dishes and top with a dollop of homemade mayonnaise.

Serves four.

Crock Pot Soups

Crock pot cooking is ideal in many ways. The food is cooked at a low temperature, vitamins and other nutrients are retained in the liquid and the cooking requires little attention from the cook. Because of the long, slow cooking time, flavors blend and marry in a way that they cannot during quick, higher heat cooking.

A soup or stew started in the morning will be ready for dinner. Start your crock pot before going to bed, and you can awaken to find a breakfast soup or stew, piping hot and ready to eat.

These recipes are designed for a four-quart crock pot and are cooked on a low temperature setting.

CELERY-LEMON SOUP

3½ cups chicken broth
8 stalks celery, thinly sliced
4 medium white potatoes, peeled and thinly sliced
6 scallions, finely chopped

3 tablespoons lemon juice
8 spinach leaves, stems removed, leaves coarsely chopped
black pepper
salt or kelp powder, to taste

Pour chicken broth into crock pot and add celery, potatoes, scallions and lemon juice. Cook for approximately 8 hours or until vegetables are tender. Use a food processor or blender to puree. Return to crock pot. Stir in seasonings to taste. Add spinach just before serving so that leaves become limp but not cooked. Freshly ground black pepper may be added at the table.

Serves four.

LIMA STEW

1 10 ounce package
  dried small lima beans
1 large Bermuda onion,
  coarsely chopped
1 clove garlic, finely
  chopped or pressed

1 turkey wing
salt or kelp powder, to
  taste
pepper, optional

Place lima beans, onion, garlic and turkey into crock pot. Fill nearly to the top with pure water. Cook for approximately 8 hours. Add seasoning if desired.

Serves six to eight.

SPLIT PEA SOUP

3½ cups split peas
2 cups sweet potatoes,
  peeled and finely
  chopped
2 cups onions, chopped

1 turkey wing, ham bone
  or other meaty bones
  for flavor
salt or kelp powder
black pepper, freshly
  ground to taste

Place all ingredients into crock pot and fill with pure water. Cook for about 8 hours. Correct seasoning if desired.

Serves six to eight.

ZUCCHINI SOUP

2½ to 3 pounds chicken
  necks
5 cups zucchini, sliced
1 cup onion, coarsely
  chopped

2 tablespoons butter
salt or kelp powder, to
  taste

Remove skin and fat from chicken necks. Place necks into a crock pot and fill with pure water. Slow cook overnight. This provides a tasty broth which is the base for this soup. Steam zucchini and onions until tender. Add onions and zucchini to 4 cups of the chicken broth. Puree in blender or food processor.

For a soup with delicate texture, blend for several minutes. For a hearty texture, blend minimally so that small bits of the vegetables remain intact.

Just before serving, heat, add butter and season to taste.

Serves six to eight.

Salads

CAULIFLOWER-BEET SALAD

1 head of cauliflower, stemmed and broken into small flowerets	salt or kelp powder
	2 cloves garlic, pressed or minced
3 tablespoons lemon juice	½ cup olive oil
	½ cup diced celery
¼ teaspoon black pepper	1 cup shredded beets

Steam cauliflower until barely tender and set aside in a bowl.

Mix lemon juice, black pepper and salt or kelp and garlic. Beat in the olive oil, adding oil slowly. This can also be done in a blender or food processor. When sauce is thick, pour it over cauliflower, raw chopped celery and shredded beets. Toss gently. Chill for a few hours before serving.

Serves four.

MINTED CUCUMBER SALAD

2 medium cucumbers,
  peeled and sliced
½ small green pepper,
  diced
2 scallions, chopped
½ cup mayonnaise
2 tablespoons lemon juice
1 clove garlic, minced or
  pressed

2 tablespoons fresh mint,
  chopped, or ½ tea-
  spoon dried mint,
  crushed
fresh mint leaves for
  garnish
lettuce leaves

Place cucumbers, pepper and scallions in a serving bowl.

In a separate bowl, mix mayonnaise, lemon juice, garlic and mint. Stir until well blended.

Add mayonnaise dressing to cucumber mixture and stir gently until vegetables are coated with dressing. Cover and chill for at least 30 minutes.

To serve from a bowl, garnish with little bunches of fresh mint leaves. To serve individually, line salad plates with fresh lettuce leaves, top with cucumber salad and garnish each plate with fresh mint leaves.

Serves four.

BROWN RICE SALAD

1 cup brown rice,
  uncooked
3 tablespoons olive oil
1 tablespoon lemon juice
¼ cup parsley, chopped
¼ cup red onion, minced
1 teaspoon Spice Island
  Italian Herb Seasoning
¼ teaspoon black pepper,
  or ⅛ teaspoon cay-
  enne pepper

salt or kelp powder, to
  taste
1 cup halved cherry
  tomatoes
½ cup green pepper,
  chopped
½ cup celery, chopped

Cook brown rice and allow to cool.

Combine olive oil, lemon juice, parsley, onion, Italian Herb Seasoning, black or cayenne pepper, and salt or kelp.

Pour dressing over rice and stir gently. Add tomatoes, chopped green pepper and chopped celery. Toss gently with brown rice. Chill for 1 to 2 hours before serving. Garnish with green pepper slices, slices of red onion and fresh parsley.

Serves four.

TURKEY SUPREME SALAD

7 or 8 asparagus stalks	2 boiled eggs, chopped
6 ounces turkey, cooked and diced	1 green onion, minced
½ pound fresh spinach, washed, stemmed and coarsely chopped	

Lightly steam asparagus and cut into 1-inch pieces. Place in a bowl with turkey, spinach, eggs and onion.

For dressing, use oil and lemon juice or add dry mustard and curry powder to mayonnaise. Pour or spoon dressing into salad and stir gently until all ingredients are coated with dressing. Chill before serving.

Serves four.

Poultry

DELECTABLE ROAST CHICKEN

1 roasting chicken	Spice Island Italian Herb Seasoning
3 cloves garlic	
4 tablespoons butter, room temperature or slightly melted	

Rinse and pat chicken dry.

Chop garlic and slide slivers of it under skin of chicken so that it is evenly distributed over breasts, near legs, etc. Place any leftover slivers of garlic inside chicken cavity.

Rub butter all over outside of chicken. Generously sprinkle Italian Herb Seasoning onto chicken. It will adhere to the butter and should coat chicken skin.

Bake in a 325° oven, basting several times. Use meat thermometer to indicate when chicken is done. The thermometer should go between the thigh and the body of the chicken without touching bone, and register 185°–190°F when chicken is done.

TURKEY WINGS ITALIAN

4 to 6 turkey wings
2 cloves garlic, pressed or minced
1 medium onion, coarsely chopped
3 cups fresh tomatoes, chopped
2 tablespoons olive oil
1 teaspoon dried basil leaves or 2 tablespoons fresh, chopped
½ teaspoon dried oregano leaves or 1 tablespoon fresh, chopped
⅛ teaspoon ground black pepper
1 bay leaf, crushed
salt or kelp powder to taste
wholegrain spaghetti or noodles, cooked immediately prior to serving

Wash and dry turkey wings. Separate at joint. Place wings, garlic and onion in a deep, heavy pot. Cover with pure water. Cover pot and simmer for 1 to 1½ hours or until wings are tender. Remove wings and add tomatoes, olive oil and seasonings to liquid. Simmer, uncovered for about 30 minutes. Add more water if needed to make sauce the desired consistency. Return turkey wings to sauce and simmer together for 5 minutes.

Serve over hot spaghetti or noodles.

Serves four.

GROUND TURKEY CHILI

2 tablespoons butter
1 clove garlic, pressed or minced
1 large onion, chopped
1 pound ground turkey
¼ cup green pepper, diced
1 teaspoon dried basil leaves or 2 tablespoons fresh, chopped

½ teaspoon dried thyme or 1 tablespoon fresh, chopped
½ teaspoon dried oregano or 1 tablespoon fresh, chopped
1 teaspoon chili powder
2 cups tomatoes, chopped
2 cups kidney beans, cooked

Heat butter on low heat in large saucepan. Sauté garlic in butter for 1 minute. Add chopped onion and cook until onions are transparent. Add turkey and green pepper and stir cook until turkey is not pink. Add all seasonings and spices, stirring well. Add tomatoes and beans and cover. Simmer for 15 to 30 minutes. Add water if needed. Serve hot.

Serves four.

CORNISH HENS WITH BULGUR WHEAT STUFFING

1 small onion, chopped
3 tablespoons butter
½ cup bulgur wheat
2 Rock Cornish hens

salt or kelp powder, to taste
black pepper, to taste

In a heavy saucepan, sauté onion in butter over low heat. When onions are tender, add bulgur wheat. Cover with water. Cover pan and simmer for 15 to 20 minutes or until tender. Add more water, if needed, during cooking process.

Rinse hens and pat dry. Rub with a little softened butter. Sprinkle with salt or kelp powder and black pepper. Spoon cooked bulgur into cavities of hens.

Bake at 325°F until tender. After hens have been removed from oven and cooled slightly, cut in half through breast with a sharp knife or poultry shears.

Garnish serving platter with bunches of fresh parsley.

Serves four.

ALL-YEAR THANKSGIVING TURKEY

6- to 8-pound turkey
(fresh is preferred. If
only frozen is avail-
able, purchase the plain
variety, not self-bast-
ing.)

Rice Giblet Dressing

Remove giblets and neck from abdominal cavity and rinse turkey well. Pat dry with paper or cotton towels. With a large spoon, stuff your turkey with the Rice Giblet Dressing on page 157. Fill the opening of the cavity by wedging in the turkey neck.

For a marvelously tender and juicy turkey, cook breast-side down in a covered earthenware roasting pan, oven temperature set at 300°F. Check after 1½ hours. When the leg joint is loose, the turkey is ready to be eaten.

This size turkey will serve 6 people with leftovers for soups, stews or salads.

Seafood

NEPTUNE'S SALAD

2 quarts boiling water
8 jumbo raw shrimps
1 lobster tail, ¾ pound
thawed
1 lemon, sliced
3 green onions, chopped
3 tablespoons olive oil

2 tablespoons fresh lime
juice
salt, optional
¼ teaspoon black pepper
1 avocado, peeled, pitted
and sliced
1 head romaine lettuce

Into boiling water drop shrimps, lobster tail and lemon. Continue to boil just until shrimps become pink. Remove shrimps. Cook lobster according to package label directions. Remove and cool in cold water. Remove shells from shrimps and lobster.

Cut lobster into ½-inch pieces and mix with shrimps in a bowl. Add chopped green onions.

In a separate bowl blend oil, lime juice, salt, if desired, and pepper. Pour over seafood and onion salad, cover and chill in refrigerator for 1 to 6 hours.

Immediately before serving add avocado to salad. For a beautiful presentation, line your salad bowl with crisp lettuce leaves and pile seafood salad into center. Serve with homemade mayonnaise to spoon over individual servings.

Serves four.

SIMPLE SCAMPI

1½ pounds extra large, raw, deveined shrimps
2 tablespoons lemon juice
1 green onion, finely chopped
2 tablespoons parsley, finely chopped
1 clove garlic, minced
4 tablespoons butter, melted
¼ cup olive oil
salt, if desired

In oven-proof casserole, combine all ingredients and toss shrimps until coated well with oil and butter mixture. Place under broiler in oven and broil the shrimps for 4 to 5 minutes on each side, basting several times with the oil and butter in the casserole. Be careful not to overcook.

Serve immediately. This is delicious served over brown rice with a tossed salad.

Serves four to six.

STEAMED ZUCCHINI AND HALIBUT

4 halibut fillets, 3 or 4
  ounces each
2 to 3 small zucchini
1 tablespoon oil
1 clove garlic, minced or
  pressed
1 teaspoon fresh ginger,
  minced

3 green onions, chopped
½ cup chicken or fish
  broth
⅛ teaspoon black pepper,
  freshly ground

Rinse fish and pat dry. Place in a buttered baking dish.

Slice zucchini into ¼-inch rounds and place rounds atop halibut in baking dish.

Heat oil on low heat and stir fry garlic, ginger and onions for 30 seconds. Add broth and pepper and bring to a simmer. Pour over fillets. Cover dish with foil or other covering and bake at 450°F for only 5 to 8 minutes. Fish should be firm to the touch. Spoon sauce over fish after serving.

Serves four.

TUNA-AVOCADO LUNCH

2 ripe avocados
1 can (6½ ounces) tuna,
  packed in water
1 small red onion,
  chopped
1 stalk celery, chopped

⅛ teaspoon cayenne
  pepper
2 tablespoons lemon juice
3 tablespoons oil
lettuce leaves

Cut avocados in half, removing pits. Brush with lemon juice to prevent them from darkening.

In a mixing bowl, mix tuna with onion and celery.

In a small bowl, mix pepper, lemon juice and oil. Pour this dressing over fish and toss. Spoon tuna mixture into avocado half.

Line dinner plates with lettuce leaves and place

avocado in center. Around avocado, arrange tomato slices, celery strips and carrot strips.

Serves four.

FISH-POTATO CASSEROLE

2 large baking potatoes, peeled and thinly sliced
1 large onion, thinly sliced
1 pound fresh or frozen fish

fresh basil, chopped
salt or kelp powder
black pepper
3 tablespoons butter

In a 1½ quart oiled casserole, layer half of the potatoes and onion slices.

Cut fish into 4 pieces. Arrange fish over vegetables and sprinkle with basil, salt, if desired, and black pepper. Melt butter and drizzle half of it over the fish and potatoes.

Layer remaining potatoes and onions over fish. Sprinkle with salt, if desired, and add more black pepper. Drizzle remaining butter over dish.

Cover and bake at 350°F for about 1 hour or until potatoes are tender and lightly browned. Sprinkle top with more chopped fresh basil leaves.

Serves four.

Meats

TARRAGON LAMB CHOPS

3 tablespoons butter
4 lamb chops
1 teaspoon dried tarragon or 2 tablespoons fresh, chopped

½ teaspoon ground black pepper
1 teaspoon salt, optional

Sauce

½ cup beef or chicken broth

1 tablespoon lemon juice

1 teaspoon dried tarragon leaves or 2 tablespoons fresh, chopped

Heat butter in a skillet over low heat and sauté lamb chops lightly. Sprinkle chops with tarragon, black pepper, and salt, if used. Cover and simmer for 15 to 20 minutes, cooking until chops are tender. Remove chops and place on platter, keeping them warm.

To prepare sauce, add broth, lemon juice and tarragon to skillet where chops cooked. Stir for 3 to 4 minutes, mixing pan drippings with other ingredients. Pour over chops just before serving.

Serves four.

LAMB STEW

2 tablespoons butter

1 pound lean lamb cubes

1 medium onion, coarsely chopped

1 garlic clove, minced or pressed

1 cup water

1 eggplant, unpeeled, cubed

1 large zucchini, cut into ½ inch thick rounds

4 fresh tomatoes, chopped

1 green pepper, sliced

3 tablespoons lemon juice

salt or kelp powder, to taste

black pepper

Over low heat, melt butter in a large kettle. Add the lamb cubes, onion and garlic. Sauté for 2 or 3 minutes. Add the water. Cover and simmer for 15 to 20 minutes. Add eggplant, zucchini, tomatoes, green pepper, lemon juice and seasonings. Stir, cover and simmer on low heat for 30 to 45 minutes or until lamb is tender.

Serves four.

INDONESIAN CURRIED BEEF

2 tablespoons butter
1 pound extra lean ground beef
1 onion, thinly sliced into rings
1 tomato, diced
1 green pepper, diced
2 tablespoons curry powder

Melt butter over low heat in a large skillet. Stir ground beef in butter until redness is gone. Add onion, tomato and green pepper. Sauté until vegetables are tender but still firm. Add curry powder. Stir well and simmer for 1 minute longer.

Serve over brown rice. Accompanying condiments may be chopped scallions and/or avocados.

Serves four.

HERBED LIVER

2 tablespoons wholewheat flour
1 teaspoon salt
⅛ teaspoon pepper
1 pound beef liver, cut into 1-inch strips
3 tablespoons butter
1 medium onion, coarsely chopped
1 clove garlic, minced or pressed
3 tablespoons parsley, minced
1 teaspoon Spice Island Italian Herb Seasoning
¼ teaspoon dry mustard
2 large tomatoes, chopped

Mix flour, salt and pepper in a paper or plastic bag. Add a few pieces of liver at a time and shake to coat.

In a large skillet with cover, melt 1 tablespoon butter over low heat. Add onion, garlic and parsley, and stir until tender. Remove from skillet. Add remaining butter and liver. Cook on low heat, stirring until lightly cooked.

Add herbs, onion mixture, mustard and tomatoes. Add a little water if needed and stir well. Bring to a boil. Simmer covered for 5 minutes, stirring once or twice.

Serve over brown rice or with steamed potatoes. Serves four.

Vegetables

ZUCCHINI PANCAKES

1 large zucchini, shredded (approximately 2 cups)
2 tablespoons onion, finely chopped
2 tablespoons wholewheat flour
¼ teaspoon salt or powdered kelp
¼ teaspoon dried oregano or 2 teaspoons fresh, chopped

1 tablespoon parsley, chopped
dash of black pepper
1 egg, beaten
butter
sprigs of parsley for garnish

In a small bowl, toss shredded zucchini and onion. Sprinkle flour, salt or kelp, oregano, parsley and black pepper on top of this mixture. Mix well with a fork and then stir in the beaten egg.

Melt a little butter in a skillet over low heat. Use about ¼ cup batter per pancake and drip onto buttered skillet. Cook on low to medium heat for 3 or 4 minutes per side. Pancakes should be golden brown and firm. Arrange on a platter, garnish with sprigs of fresh parsley and serve while still hot.

Makes 8 small pancakes.

EGGPLANT STICKS

1 eggplant
½ cup butter
¼ cup onion, grated

2 cloves garlic, minced or pressed
salt, if desired

Peel and cut eggplant lengthwise into slender strips. Arrange strips on a greased baking dish.

Melt butter and add onion and garlic. Brush butter mixture onto eggplant sticks.

Broil eggplant for 5 minutes. Turn, brush with remaining butter mixture and broil for another 5 minutes.

Serve immediately. Season with salt, if desired.

Serves four.

STUFFED PEPPERS

4 large green peppers
1 cup onion, chopped
1 medium tomato, chopped
1 stick celery, chopped
¼ cup parsley, chopped
¼ teaspoon Spice Island Italian Herb Seasoning

2 tablespoons butter
1 cup brown rice, leftover or freshly cooked
salt or kelp powder
black pepper

Wash peppers. Cut off tops so that you can use them as covers while baking. Remove seeds from inside peppers. Steam peppers and tops until barely tender.

Sauté chopped vegetables and herbs in melted butter over low heat. Stir in rice and seasonings with salt or kelp and pepper to taste.

Place peppers in a buttered baking dish. Fill with rice mixture and replace tops of peppers. Bake, uncovered, at 350°F until heated thoroughly.

Serves four.

HARDY LENTIL STEW

2 tablespoons butter
4 medium potatoes, chopped
3 medium onions, chopped
1 clove garlic, minced or pressed
1 cup carrots, sliced
1 cup celery, chopped
1 red pepper, chopped
1½ cups brown dried lentils

1½ cups tomatoes, peeled and diced
1 quart pure water
2 small bay leaves
1 teaspoon dried basil leaves or 2 table- spoons fresh, chopped
chopped parsley

In a large casserole or pot, melt butter over low heat. Add potatoes, onions and garlic and cook briefly. Add carrots, celery and red pepper, cooking for a few minutes. Add all other ingredients, stir well and simmer, covered, for about 1 hour. Stir occasionally and add more water if needed.

Serves six.

Grains

Freshly cooked whole grains can substitute for the yeasty bread that you will not be eating on your anti-Candida diet. These grains can be purchased in health food stores, specialty sections of fine super- markets and from co-ops.

Millet

In many parts of the world, this grain is a staple in the diet. Here, in the U.S.A., we know it as bird seed! Millet doesn't have to be for the birds. It is a delicious, nutritious, complex carbohydrate.

Don't buy millet in a pet store as this type is unwhole and unfit for human consumption. Millet sold for people to eat has the hard hull removed.

½ cup millet
2 cups pure water

butter
salt, if desired

Soak millet for 6 to 8 hours in water. Simmer over low heat, covered, for 15 to 20 minutes. When cooked, millet will be light, fluffy and soft. Add butter and salt, if desired, before serving.

Bulgur Wheat

Bulgur is a precooked, cracked wheat. It is very much like brown rice and can be used in many ways that rice is used. It has a pleasant nutty taste and requires little cooking. It can be used in salads, added to soups, and included in casseroles.

PILAF

2 tablespoons butter
1 tablespoon onion, chopped
1 cup bulgur

2 cups water or chicken broth
½ teaspoon salt or kelp powder

Melt butter in a skillet over low heat. Add onion and sauté for a few minutes. Add bulgur wheat and stir cook over low heat until the color becomes golden brown.

Add water or chicken broth and seasonings. Cover and bring to a simmer, cooking for about 15 minutes. Serves four.

Brown Rice

Brown rice is far superior to white rice in almost every way. It has more vitamins, minerals and fiber. Once you become accustomed to its rich, nutty flavor, you will find white rice bland and insipid.

RICE GIBLET DRESSING

2½ cups pure water
2 turkey or chicken livers, chopped
2 turkey or chicken gizzards, chopped
1 turkey or chicken heart, chopped

½ cup onion, chopped
1 cup celery, chopped
1 clove garlic, minced or pressed
1½ cups brown rice
½ teaspoon salt

Bring water to a boil. Add chopped poultry organs and reduce to low heat. Cover and allow to simmer while you chop the onions, celery and garlic.

Add the chopped vegetables to the simmering broth and bring this mixture to a boil. Once it is boiling, add brown rice. Stir in ½ teaspoon salt. Reduce to low heat, cover and allow to simmer for about 30 minutes.

If you wish to use this recipe for stuffing a turkey or other poultry, use half the amount of water and cook the rice for only 15 minutes. Then stuff the poultry cavity with the partially cooked rice dressing and allow it to complete its cooking along with the poultry.

Dessert

What? A dessert on an anti-Candida diet!

While desserts are the rare exception, not the rule on a pro-human, healing diet, this recipe will provide you with an occasional treat that is not stressful to body chemistry.

SWEET POTATO SOUFFLÉ

6 cups sweet potatoes,
peeled and cubed
3 eggs, separated into
yolks and whites
1 teaspoon pumpkin pie
spice

1 package unflavored
gelatin
¼ cup pure water
1 pint whipping cream

Steam sweet potatoes until tender. Spoon into a large mixing bowl and mash until no lumps remain. Add egg yolks and pumpkin pie spice and mix.

Dissolve gelatin into heated pure water and add to sweet potato mixture. Blend well.

In a small mixing bowl, beat egg whites until stiff. Gently fold egg whites into the sweet potato mixture. This will result in a light, soufflé-like texture. Pour into a 9-inch pie dish and refrigerate immediately. For a more traditional dessert, line the pie plate with your favorite wholegrain crust.

Serve with a dollop of unsweetened whipped cream.

REFERENCES

Benson, H. *Beyond the Relaxation Response*. New York: Times Books, 1984.

Bundy, P. K. *Diseases of Metabolism*. Philadelphia: W. B. Saunders Co., 1969.

Cheraskin, E., W.M. Ringsdorf, Jr., E. Sisley. *The Vitamin C Connection*. New York: Harper and Row, 1982.

Cheraskin, E., W.M. Ringsdorf, Jr., R.R. Ramsay, Jr. "Sucrose, Neutrophilic Phagocytosis and Resistance to Disease." *Dental Survey* (1976) 52: 46–48.

Cousins, N. *Anatomy of an Illness*. New York: W.W. Norton & Co., Inc. 1979.

Crook, W.C. *The Yeast Connection*. Jackson, TN: Professional Books, 1984.

Galton, L. "Finally Help For Fungus Disease." *Parade* (June 13, 1982).

Garrison, R. H., E. Somer. *The Nutrition Desk Reference*. New Canaan, CT.: Keats Pub., Inc. 1985.

Gaul, J. W. "The Rule of the Artery." *Let's Live* (October 1979).

Graham, T.M. *Biology—the Essential Principles*. Philadelphia: W. B. Saunders Press, 1982.

Hickman, F.M. *Biological Science—an Inquiry Into Life*. New York: Harcourt Brace Jovanovich, Inc., 1980.

Jenson, W.A., F. B. Salisbury. *Botany, an Ecological Approach*. Belmont, CA: Wadsworth, Inc., 1972.

Kimbau, J.W. *Biology*. Reading, Massachusetts: Addison-Wesley Pub., Co., Inc., 1968.

Langer, S.E. *Solved: the Riddle of Illness*. New Canaan, CT: Keats Pub., Inc., 1984.

Long, J. W. *The Essential Guide to Prescription Drugs.* New York: Harper & Row, 1982.

Mader, S. S. *Inquiry Into Life.* Dubuque, Iowa: William C. Group, 1979.

McKegney, F. P. "Psychoneuroimmunology: What Lies Ahead." *Drug Therapy* (August 1982) 159–166.

Page, M. E., H. L. Abrams, Jr. *Your Body Is Your Best Doctor.* New Canaan, CT: Keats Pub. Inc., 1972.

Page, M. E. *Degeneration Regeneration.* St. Petersburg, FL: Nutritional Development, 1949.

Pfeiffer, C. C. *Mental and Elemental Nutrients.* New Canaan, CT: Keats Pub. Inc., 1975.

Raab, W. *The Treatment of Mycosis with Imidazole Derivatives.* Berlin: Springer-Verlag, 1980.

Rippon, J. W. *Medical Mycology.* Philadelphia: W. B. Saunders Press, 1982.

Sanchez, A., et al. "Role of Sugars in Human Neutrophilic Phagocytosis." *The American Journal of Clinical Nutrition* 26:1180–1184.

Schauss, A. *Diet, Crime and Delinquency.* Berkeley: Parker House, 1981.

Sherman, I.W., V. G. Sherman. *Biology, a Human Approach.* New York: Oxford University Press, 1979.

Taheebo, "An Herb for All Reasons." *Spotlight Newspaper* Washington, D.C.

Truss, C. O. *The Missing Diagnosis.* Birmingham, AL: C. Orian Truss, M.D., 1982.

Truss, C. O. "Tissue Injury Induced by Candida Albicans; Mental and Neurological Manifestations." *The Journal of Orthomolecular Psychiatry.* (1978) 7:17–37.

Truss, C. O. "Restoration of Immunologic Competence to Candida Albicans." *The Journal of Orthomolecular Psychiatry* (1980) 9:287–301.

Truss, C. O. "The Role of Candida Albicans in Illness." *The Journal of Orthomolecular Psychiatry* (1981) 10:228–238.

Villee, Z. *Biology.* Philadelphia: W. B., Saunders Co., 1972.

Walker, M. *The Chelation Answer.* New York: M. Evans & Co., Inc. 1982.

Wallace, A. *Biology, the World of Life,* Santa Monica, CA: Goodyear Pub. Co., Inc., 1981.

References

Winchester, A. M. *Biology and Its Relation to Mankind.* New York: Van Nostrand Reinhold Pub. Co., Inc. 1975.

Zamm, A. V. *Why Your House May Endanger Your Health.* New York: Simon & Schuster, Inc., 1980.

Ziff, S. *Silver Dental Fillings, the Toxic Time Bomb.* New York: Aurora Press, 1984.

INDEX

INDEX

Index